The Safe Baby

A Do-It-Yourself Guide to Home Safety and Healthy Living

Third Edition

DEBRA SMILEY HOLTZMAN

SENTIENT PUBLICATIONS

For Robert, Julian, Laura, Jonathan,
Adam, Samantha and baby Emma.

In the blessed memory of my parents:
Harriet and Irving Smiley.

───────────

Library of Congress Cataloging-in-Publication Data
Names: Holtzman, Debra Smiley, author.
Title: The safe baby : a do-it-yourself guide to home safety and healthy living / Debra Smiley Holtzman.
Description: Third edition. | Boulder, CO : Sentient Publications, 2018. | Includes index.
Identifiers: LCCN 2018001478 (print) | LCCN 2018001541 (ebook) | ISBN 9781591812999 | ISBN 9781591812906
Subjects: LCSH: Home accidents--Prevention.
Classification: LCC TX150 (ebook) | LCC TX150 .H652 2018 (print) | DDC 363.13/7—dc23
LC record available at https://lccn.loc.gov/2018001478
Printed in the United States of America
10 9 8 7 6 5 4 3 2 1

SENTIENT PUBLICATIONS
A Limited Liability Company
PO Box 7204
Boulder, CO 80304
www.sentientpublications.com

Contents

Acknowledgments

I especially thank my editor, Drollene P. Brown; my agent, Pamela Harty, of The Knight Agency; Connie Shaw and the staff at Sentient Publications; my husband, Robert Holtzman, M.D.; and my sisters, Madeleine Levy, Karen Pollack and Dr. Elena Holtzman.

Thanks to the many organizations and governmental agencies, and the people who spoke for them, who promptly and graciously answered my inquires, supplied me with information, or reviewed sections of the book: Centers for Disease Control and Prevention; Food and Drug Administration; Consumer Product Safety Commission; National Highway Traffic Safety Administration; USDA Meat and Poultry Hotline; Environmental Working Group; Florida Department of Health; Florida Department of Health Radon Program staff; Bob Vincent, R.S., M.P.A., Water Programs, Florida Dept. of Health; American Academy of Pediatrics; National Center on Shaken Baby Syndrome, especially Ryan Steinbeigle; Dr. Toby Litovitz, M.D., and Nicole Reid of the National Capital Poison Center; Safe to Sleep® Campaign of the Eunice Kennedy Shriver National Institute of Child Health and Human Development of the National Institutes of Health; Kids in Danger, especially Nancy A. Cowles; Brady Center to Prevent Gun Violence; National Shooting Sports Foundation, especially Bill Brassard, Jr.; SafetyBeltSafe U.S. A., especially Stephanie Tombrello; Kansas State University Radon Programs, especially Brian Hanson; National Program for Playground Safety, especially Donna Thompson, Ph.D.; National Fire Protection Administration, especially Lisa Braxton; Judy Bannon, Cribs for Kids; Linda Kaiser, Parents for Window Blind Safety; Joyce Davis, Keeping Babies Safe.

For reviewing sections of the book and providing information, thanks to Pam Borchardt, Borchardt Consulting; Mario Vittone, Water Safety Expert; Judy Towne Jennings, PT, MA; Brian D. Johnston MD MPH; Monte Levy ; and Dr. Neil Pollack of Brookhaven Country Day Camp.

A special thanks to my colleagues in Florida for answering all my questions, reviewing sections of the book, and supplying information: Teresa Brevda, RN, FACCE; Nirvanni Chatoori, PhD, RNC-MNN, LE-C; Sue Englund, RN, BSN; Mark Rubin, President, Xact, Natural Pest Management; Cecilia Haroon; Justina Supple; Mark Horowitz; Alan D. Mendelsohn M.D., F.A.C.S.; and buybuy BABY Coral Springs.

Introduction

B ecause we live in a changing world, a child safety book is only as successful as its latest edition. *The Safe Baby* has had two editions that parents, grandparents and other adults who care for children found abundantly helpful. But since the second edition came out in 2009, a lot of new information has come to the forefront. Now I've brought all the latest, best guidance I could find and added it to *The Safe Baby* in this third edition.

As our world has changed, it has become, in some respects, more dangerous. In addition, the economy seems to have shrunk for many of us, and budgets have necessarily become tighter. Now, more than ever, we have to find clever ways to solve problems instead of simply buying products. We have to make choices, and sometimes, in doing so, we must weigh both safety and economy. A new parent can laugh at the "old days" when "Paper or plastic?" was the biggest question of the day. With a baby in the house, you are asking, plastic bottles or glass? What shampoos, sunscreens and detergents are safe for my baby? Is the brand sold on discount as safe as the brand touted on TV?

The first edition of *The Safe Baby* primarily addressed safety concerns. The second edition added tips that addressed ways to stretch the dollars in your wallet. This edition will keep those elements and add some new topics, as well as introducing new federal safety standards for nursery products such as cribs, bassinets, play yards and strollers.

The Safe Baby third edition keeps all the good information from the first two books about do-it-yourself projects and room-by-room inspections to make them safe for baby, but there are some great new topics and resources: "Ten Steps to Mindfulness Meditation," "Supervise

Children's Media Use," and "Tips for New Grandparents." And there are lots of little tweaks to other chapters in the book.

One thing that never changes is the opinion of folks who think the way they used to do things is good enough for now. You probably won't have to worry about Uncle Bill wanting to smoke in the house, but he may see nothing wrong with smoking on your porch or patio while his little niece is sitting beside him. And Aunt Ethel may insist on your using the crib she's passed down from cousin to cousin. Don't give in to get along. You will learn a lot about safety as you read this book; stick to the best safety and health practices for your baby.

Having told you to follow my advice, I'd like you to know that you can cut yourself some slack. The last thing I want is for parents to be overwhelmed with all these dos and don'ts. You'll get lots of facts here to help you keep your child safe, but the greatest safety is found in your love. With your love will come the vigilance that I write so much about; you can watch without making yourself and your child nervous wrecks. Remember this: you don't have to do everything perfectly to usher your child into adulthood. Have fun with your baby! These are precious years.

If you have questions not covered in this book, I invite you to contact me in any of the following venues:

- TheSafetyExpert.com
- facebook.com/DebraHoltzmanTheSafetyExpert
- Twitter.com/safetyexpert_

I'm always eager to learn your concerns and read your comments. In fact, they will help me plan the next edition of this book!

TIPS FOR
NEW GRANDPARENTS AND OTHERS
WHO DID IT DIFFERENTLY AND
THEIR KIDS TURNED OUT JUST FINE

Remember When

Back in the day you used paint that stunk to high heaven, and it didn't kill anybody. Why pay more for special eco-friendly paint? (Did you notice whether anyone in the family felt a little queasy for a few days after the painting? Did anyone have a headache?)

You've never heard of the off-gassing of new carpet. You bought the carpet, rolled it out, and installed it in the room. Sure, it stinks, but a little smell never hurt anyone. (Are you sure about that? Have you ever noticed feeling a little sick from the smell?) And think about a closed nursery with these types of smells permeating the area ... as well as the eyes, nose and throat of an infant.

When you and your children were growing up, most kids biked and skated without helmets and knee pads and elbow guards. You may be thinking we probably had a lot more fun, too. (But weren't there a lot of scrapes and bruises, and weren't there a few runs to the emergency room? Wouldn't you like to protect your little loved one from that kind of trauma?)

You didn't put guards on electric sockets when your children were small—never heard of 'em. That's just overdoing the safety bit. (But how many children do you know who stuck a hairpin or a key into a wall socket? Did the child get a painful burn? Why take a chance now when electrical outlet covers are so easy to buy?) *continues*

(CONTINUED) TIPS FOR NEW GRANDPARENTS AND OTHERS WHO DID IT DIFFERENTLY AND THEIR KIDS TURNED OUT JUST FINE

Get With The Times

You know very well that times have changed. You wouldn't think of allowing your grandchildren—or great-grandchildren—to wander about the neighborhood unsupervised the way you did when you were a child. The world is not a safe place. You don't need a book to tell you that. However, there are some safety issues about which you may not be aware, and I'm hoping you will read through my entire book to learn more about what we've discovered about keeping our children safe.

Grandparents make very special contributions to the lives of their grandchildren, but you must recognize that things have changed significantly in the child safety and health arena. There is new knowledge about proper sleep position, crib safety and car seat use since your own children were born. There are new products—safer paints, detectors for poisonous gases, protective gear and gadgets to make the home safer. And, of course, you do want your adult children to have trust and confidence in your abilities to safely care for your grandchildren and to provide a safe environment when they come to visit. It's easy to get up to speed to equip grandparents with the latest up-to-date skills and tools. You can attend an infant/ child first aid and CPR course, and you can read *The Safe Baby*

Your wisdom is also important, but knowing when and where to impart that wisdom is probably the most difficult part of loving a child while not being the parent. Maintaining boundaries and avoiding giving advice when it is not requested is hard, hard, hard! Here's a friendly bit of advice for family harmony dynamics: It really doesn't matter who you are—even if you're a baby safety expert or a trauma surgeon. Advice and opinions on child rearing are generally not welcomed by adult children unless they directly solicit it and really want to hear what you have to share. The best policy is to zip the lip. Let your children make their own decisions and be in charge of parenting. And never say, "We didn't do it that way, and our kids turned out just fine."

Part I

Room to Room for Safety

In Part I we'll consider three specific rooms in the home, the ones in which your little darling may well spend the most time at first: nursery (Chapter 1), kitchen (Chapters 2 and 3), and bathroom (Chapter 4). It will be obvious to you that some of the same guidelines are to be followed in other rooms, as well. But I don't have to tell *you* that—after all, you're a do-it-yourselfer. Remember previous tips when you walk into the living room or out in the yard.

Creating a Safe Nursery

The nursery is where the new baby will spend most of his time. I'm sure you'll want to decorate the room beautifully, giving it lots of little touches that will make it a pleasant place. While you are doing this, you'll want to make safety your first priority. Safety is your top concern when it comes to your baby and your home. That's why we're beginning this book by discussing ways to make the nursery safe. (In addition to this chapter, there is information about keeping the nursery safe from chemicals in Chapter 11, "Environmental Hazards.")

More than 3,500 babies in the U.S. die suddenly and unexpectedly every year while sleeping, often due to sudden infant death syndrome (SIDS) or accidental deaths from suffocation or strangulation, according to the American Academy of Pediatrics (AAP).

You can take simple precautions to reduce the risk of all sleep-related deaths.

Choose the Right Crib and Mattress

The most important piece of furniture you will buy for your child is her crib, so be especially vigilant when choosing it, keeping in mind that *safety is the crib's most important feature.*

If possible, purchase a new crib. A secondhand one may have missing or broken parts, be weak with age, have lead paint, or have an unsafe design. In addition, a used crib is not likely to have the manufacturer's instructions, and worse, it may have been recalled. Do not use a crib made before June 28, 2011, because it will not meet current safety standards. The new federal safety standards prohibit the manufacture or sale of drop-side rail cribs. But drop-sides are not the only significant changes: the regulations also require that all cribs have stronger slats and mattress supports and better quality hardware, and they have to have undergone more rigorous testing. I'm happy to say that the United States has the strongest crib safety standards in the world.

As you shop for your baby's new crib, make sure the product has a label stating that it meets Consumer Product Safety Commission (CPSC) standards. In addition, look for the Juvenile Products Manufacturers Association (JPMA) certification label. If your circumstances dictate that you must buy or accept a secondhand crib, be sure to test it according to the guidelines in the sidebar. Carefully read the instructions for setup and use of the crib. (If the instructions have been misplaced, replacement instructions can be obtained from the manufacturer.) If you aren't certain how to assemble a new crib correctly, ask the retailer to send a qualified person to your home.

If the secondhand crib you have does not meet the checklist guidelines, it should be destroyed, or at least completely modified, so that no one will consider putting a baby in it. (Creative folk may turn the rails into a flower bed...just don't let your toddler get into it!) You can also take the wood, plastic, and metal from the crib to recycling centers. The mattress however, must be consigned to a waste disposal center.

You will learn in this chapter and throughout the book that a surprising number of items you thought you needed you actually don't need. Some of these are things you should not buy for safety reasons. The money you save by not buying these items can be used to buy a new crib.

It is always best to buy a new, firm mattress. For sanitary reasons, I do not recommend a used mattress, but whether new or used, the mattress you choose should be as firm as possible and not covered with any soft padding. When shopping for a mattress, press your hand firmly into it. If there is an indentation when you take your hand away, the mattress is not firm enough. Your handprint on the mattress indicates that it will indent when your baby is lying on it, and that could be life-threatening for your child. If the mattress has a soft side and a firm side, use the firm side for the infant. The softer side is intended for use in a toddler bed with an older child.

The mattress you select should fit tightly in the crib. You must not be able to put two fingers between the mattress and crib sides. Baby can suffocate if his head or body becomes wedged between the mattress and the crib sides.

DO IT YOURSELF!

Make your crib meet the safety test by matching it with each description.

- The crib has not been recalled by the CSPC. (See Appendix D, "Recall Information" to learn how to check for recalled products. Millions of cribs have been recalled in past years.)
- There is no missing, loose, damaged or improperly installed hardware, including screws, bolts, or brackets on the crib or mattress support.
- Slats are no more than 2 3/8 inches apart. If you are able to pass a soda can between the slats, they are too far apart. The baby's head could get caught.
- Post extensions at the corners of the crib are less than 1/16 of an inch high. Larger extensions can cause entanglement.
- There are no cutouts in the head- or footboard. The baby's head could get stuck there, too.
- The mattress fits snugly into the crib. You must not be able to put two fingers between the mattress and crib sides. Baby can suffocate if his head or body becomes wedged between the mattress and the crib sides.
- The mattress support hangers are secured to the crib frame with bolts or closed hooks.
- The crib is smooth. There is no cracked or peeling paint, all painted surfaces are lead-free, and the crib has no splinters, rough edges or other defects.
- The crib was manufactured after June 28, 2011. If the sides go down, don't use the crib!

Reduce the Risk of Sudden Infant Death Syndrome

Sudden infant death syndrome (SIDS) is the sudden, unexplained death of an infant under 1 year of age. It is more common among premature and low birth-weight babies and among twins and triplets. Slightly more boys die of SIDS than girls.

Recent studies indicate that there may be an abnormality in the brain stems of many SIDS victims that makes them vulnerable to sudden, unexpected deaths. Things that a healthy baby can overcome, such as rebreathing carbon dioxide, overheating, and exposure to secondhand smoke, can be fatal to a baby predisposed with this brain stem abnormality. Currently there is no way to detect this abnormality.

While the cause of SIDS is still not definitive and SIDS may not always be preventable, we can take precautions. Since the beginning of a campaign called "Back to Sleep"—which recommends that babies be placed on their backs and all soft bedding be removed from their cribs—SIDS rates have dropped more than 50 percent and these precautions will 100% eliminate the risk of accidental suffocation.

The subject of SIDS brings us right back to crib safety and a few more necessary discussion points. The current recommendations for infant safe sleep and guidelines for reducing the likelihood of a sleep-related death are:

- Put your baby on his back to sleep at night and naptime until the child reaches one year of age. Research shows that the back-sleep position carries the lowest risk of SIDS. Putting your baby to sleep on his back also helps prevent suffocation. Don't worry that a baby who sleeps on his back will choke if he spits up during sleep. According to the American Academy of Pediatrics, babies' airway anatomy and gag reflex will prevent them from choking while sleeping on their backs.
- Remove soft objects and loose bedding from the sleep area. This includes bumpers, pillows, blankets, quilts, sheepskins, sleep positioners, stuffed toys, and any other soft products or extra padding. The reason for this is that when the baby sleeps on her tummy or there is soft bedding in or around her sleep area, carbon dioxide (exhaled air) can build up around her head and face. Instead of breathing fresh air, she rebreathes this bad air. Rebreathing carbon dioxide has been identified as a leading cause of sudden infant deaths. In addition, soft bedding can block a baby's airway during sleep. In fact, the only things that should be in the crib are a firm, snugly fitting mattress, a tight-fitting sheet, and the baby. (See information about bumpers and sleep positioners in a later section.) Remember, bare is best. The crib is the only place where baby is left unattended for hours at a time. This is baby's sleep place, not a play place.
- Use crib sheets that fit securely on all corners and sides. Check carefully for shrinkage after each wash. A child can pull poorly fitted sheets loose and become entrapped.
- Don't hang anything on or above the crib with a ribbon or string longer than 7 inches.

- Position any mobile or hanging crib toy out of your child's reach. This means that any such toy or crib gym must be removed when the baby begins to push up on his hands and knees, or when the baby is 5 months old, whichever comes first. These toys can strangle a baby. Any pieces the baby may pull off the mobile can present a choking hazard.
- Don't put the baby to sleep on a waterbed, sofa, couch, arm chair, air mattress, soft mattress, pillow, or any other soft surface. These are designed for adults, not infants.
- Don't let your baby sleep in a car seat, carrier, swing, bouncy chair or anything like them. These are not safe for sleeping babies. When your baby falls asleep, always place him on his back in his crib. (Note: It's OK for baby to sleep in a properly installed car seat while the car is moving. When the car seat is taken out of the car, the pitch changes and makes it unsafe for a young infant to sleep because they do not have the neck strength to keep their airway open.)
- Don't let your baby overheat during sleep. Keep the room temperature and your baby's clothing at what would be comfortable for a lightly clothed adult. AAP recommends: in general dress your baby in no more than one extra layer than you would wear. Your baby may be too hot if she is sweating or if her chest feels hot. If you are worried that your baby is cold, use a wearable blanket, such as a sleep sack, or warm sleeper that is the right size for your baby, as a safe alternative to loose blankets.
- See that the baby's head and face remain uncovered while he is asleep.
- *Room Sharing, Not Bed Sharing.* Placing the baby's crib or bassinet near your bed is safer than bed sharing. A baby should not share a bed, sofa, couch or armchair with an adult or other child. Experts have serious concerns about potentially hazardous conditions present in the family bed or sofa (such as pillows, comforters, and other bodies). Moreover, bed sharing has not been found to be protective against SIDS. Room sharing (having baby nearby) reduces the risk of SIDS by as much as 50%. It's okay to bring the baby into bed for nursing or comforting, but it is important to return the baby to his own separate space when you're ready to sleep. If you bring your baby into your bed for feeding or comforting, remove all soft items and bedding from the area. When finished, put

baby back in the crib or bassinet. Keeping baby in your room and close to your bed for at least the first 6 months is recommended.

Important Note: Couches and armchairs are extremely dangerous for babies, as they pose an extraordinarily high risk of infant death, including SIDS and suffocation, if adults fall asleep as they feed, comfort or bond with baby while on these surfaces. Therefore, parents and other caregivers should be especially vigilant of how tired they are during these times, warns the American Academy of Pediatrics.

- Do not allow smoking anywhere near your baby! Babies who are exposed to tobacco, either during pregnancy or after birth, are at increased risk for SIDS. The more significant the exposure, the higher the risk. You will find more information on secondhand smoke in Chapter 11, "Environmental Hazards."
- Consider offering your baby a clean, dry pacifier every time you put her down to sleep for the first year of her life. Recent research has shown that pacifiers can reduce a baby's risk for SIDS. It is not necessary to put the pacifier back if it falls out—she is still protected, once she falls asleep. If you are breastfeeding, wait until nursing is well established (usually one month) before offering a pacifier. If your baby refuses the pacifier after a few weeks of trying, do not force it. We don't know for sure why pacifiers reduce risk, but experts think it may be because it helps keep the airway open or because it prevents the baby from falling into a deep sleep, which can be dangerous. Do not use pacifiers that attach to infant clothing or to objects such as stuffed toys and other items that may be a suffocation or choking risk.
- Educate anyone who cares for your baby about these important tips. Give them a list of guidelines to follow and stress how important they are. Some caregivers (especially grandparents) are not aware of the new rules about back sleeping and soft bedding. Consistency in care is critical to safe sleep for baby. Babies who are used to sleeping in a safe environment and are suddenly placed on their tummy or near soft bedding are at a much higher risk to die suddenly and unexpectedly. Make sure your baby has a safe place to sleep for naps and at nighttime, at home and everywhere else, and make sure others who care for him follow your rules.

To maximize your baby's health, take her for regular checkups and follow her immunization schedule. If your baby seems ill, contact the pediatrician immediately. Breast-feed your baby; breast milk contains nutrients and antibodies that are needed to help keep your baby healthy. (Babies who breastfeed, or are fed breast milk in a bottle, are at lower risk for SIDS than babies who were never fed breast milk. The longer a baby is exclusively breastfed or fed breast milk, the lower the risk.) Take preventive measures during pregnancy: do not smoke while pregnant; do not drink alcohol or take any drugs not prescribed for you by your physician after you become pregnant; go for frequent medical checkups; and eat nutritious meals. This kind of care helps keep your baby from having problems that could put her at risk for SIDS.

An additional caution comes from the AAP: Do not rely on home heart or breathing monitors to reduce the risk of SIDS. If you have questions about using these monitors for other health conditions, talk with your pediatrician.

There's something else to note in terms of parental behavior: When your baby starts to turn himself over—at about 5 months—you don't have to stay up all night checking on him. Continue to put him down to sleep on his back and get some sleep yourself! SIDS occurs most often in infants 2 to 4 months of age, and 90% of SIDS victims are under 6 months of age. The important thing is that your baby start every sleep time on his back to reduce the risk of SIDS, and that there are no soft objects, toys, bumpers, or loose bedding under baby, over baby, or anywhere in baby's sleep area. Research suggests that the prime developmental step for your baby's safe sleep is rolling. Once a baby can roll freely (back to front and front to back), place baby on her back to sleep but allow her to adopt whatever position that she prefers.

Additional Precautions as Baby Grows Older

Before your baby can stand up, adjust the mattress to the lowest position.

When your child makes a habit of climbing out of the crib or when she is 35 inches tall, that is the time for a toddler "big-kid" bed.

As long as your baby sleeps in the crib—regardless of whether it is new or used—periodically inspect it for missing hardware, chipped or peeled paint, holes and tears, loose threads, and strings.

Use Crib Rules as You Select Other Nursery Furniture

Bassinets or cradles are smaller sleep environments used for younger infants. When selecting a bassinet, be sure that it was manufactured on

---

FOLLOW THE ABCs OF
SAFE SLEEP FOR INFANTS

Alone: Infants should always sleep or nap alone without siblings or other people.

Back: Always put a baby on his back to sleep or nap until he is a year old.

Crib: Babies should always sleep or nap in a safety-approved crib, bassinet or play yard that meets CPSC and JPMA Standards.

Remember: When it comes to baby's sleep environment, bare really is best!

---

or after April 23, 2014, so it will meet current standards. Look for the JPMA certification. Always follow manufacturer recommendations for age and weight in order to know when to move a baby up to a crib. The same safety precautions apply to bassinets, cradles and play yards as they do to cribs. (See chapter 5, "Preventing Falls in the Home," for more information about play yard safety.)

Choose all the furniture in your baby's room with care, and use the rules you've learned about the crib to help you select other pieces. Be as wary in accepting other used products for the nursery as you are in accepting a used crib. Make sure the furniture is sturdy, with no loose, missing or improperly installed parts, no chipped paint, and no rough, sharp edges. Check that the materials have no tears or holes. Take away any ties or loops. Make sure the item meets current national safety standards. Look for the JPMA label, and check with the CPSC to make sure it hasn't been recalled. You'll learn more about recalled products in Chapter 5, "Preventing Falls in the Home." We'll talk about ways to make ordinary furniture safer when we move to other rooms in the house.

Consider Investing in a Baby Monitor

Now that your baby has a safe crib and safe furniture, can you be sure he is completely safe when you leave him alone in the room? You can't stay in the nursery all the time, so consider investing in a baby monitor and keep it on any time the child is alone in the room. (Be sure to place baby monitors, cameras, and cords at least 3 feet away from any part of the crib, bassinet, or play yard.)

DO IT YOURSELF!

Make a safe zone around the crib, bassinet, and play yard.
To help reduce the risk of falls, strangulation, suffocation, and burns, create a safety zone—at least 3 feet—around the crib, bassinet, and play yard.
Do not position near windows, draperies, window covering cords, electrical cords, baby monitor cords and other cords, hanging wall decorations, heating sources, or climbable furniture.

Every family is different, so when choosing a monitor you must consider your budget as well as your needs. The simplest monitor is the audio-only device. If you choose this option, Digital Enhanced Cordless Technology (DECT) is recommended over analog systems. DECT encrypts the transmission to prevent others from listening in.

A video monitor can add another dimension to your ability to keep tabs on what is happening in the nursery while you are in another room. A night vision camera is yet another feature you may like if you wish to watch your baby sleep in a darkened room, but it should not add cost; this feature is standard for most video monitors.

A step up from those monitors is a Wi-Fi connected video monitor that can send a live video feed to your smartphone, tablet or laptop. These are only accessible with a user name and password and parents can restrict the viewing access from an administrative account. A Wi-Fi system must be in place at the home. There are also smart home security cameras that can send a video feed to any of those devices via an app. If you use a Wi-Fi connected baby monitor or camera, keep its firmware updated, along with your router's firmware and security features.

However, even if you have the newest, best monitor money can buy, nothing takes the place of checking on your child in person, to make sure everything is okay. Peek in once in a while to give yourself a smile.

Consider Carefully Your Choice of a Diaper Pail

One piece of essential equipment that may seem incidental is the diaper pail. When you get one, make sure it has a locking lid. A child can drown in the accumulated liquid in the pail. If deodorizers are used, keep them out of the reach of children. Once your child is getting around on his own, he may try to eat them, and some are poisonous. (Remember to wash your hands after each diaper change.)

Be Safe: Products to Avoid

Bumpers

Crib bumpers are linked to serious injuries and deaths from suffocation, strangulation and entrapment.

In addition, the bumper may restrict the movement of fresh air in the crib. Also, bumpers can be used by your baby to launch herself out of the crib once she is able to pull up and stand.

You may need to explain to your mother or Aunt Sue why bumper pads may have seemed necessary when you or Cousin Judy were infants but are no longer needed for a baby's safety. Here's what to tell them: Before crib safety was regulated, the spacing between the slats of the crib sides could be any width; when the spaces between slats were too wide, babies could be injured by getting between the slats. Now that cribs must meet strict safety standards, the slats don't pose the same dangers.

If you are concerned that, in the absence of a bumper, if your baby rolls into the side of the crib he will sustain a bruise or injury to his head, you should understand that this is an unlikely occurrence. While it is true that a child's arms or legs can get stuck in the slats, serious injury is improbable. Moreover, a child can get an arm or leg stuck under or above a bumper.

Legislation has begun to catch up with acknowledging the dangers of bumper pads. In April of 2012, Chicago became the first city in the U.S. to ban the sale of crib bumper pads. In 2013, Maryland followed suit, becoming the first state to ban these dangerous products. More recently, both the state of Ohio and the borough of Watchung, New Jersey, also banned non-mesh crib bumper pads.

Sleep Positioners

Sleep positioners are devices claimed by their manufacturers to help keep baby on his back and reduce the risk of SIDS. The two most common types of sleep positioners feature raised supports or pillows (called "bolsters") that are attached to each side of a mat, or a wedge to raise a baby's head. These products have never proven to prevent SIDS and since they are generally made out of soft materials they pose a suffocation hazard to your baby. The American Academy of Pediatrics, The FDA, and the CPSC and other safety organizations warn against using these products because of the dangers that pose to babies. Many of these products are associated with injury and death, especially when used in baby's sleep area.

Avoiding Common Hazards

Prevent Shocks and Burns

When an electrical outlet is not in use, cover it! Take care when you choose the outlet plugs. Your little explorer may find a way to pull one out . . . and when the plug comes out, it will go directly into his mouth. Then he is in danger of choking, as well as getting a bad burn. The lesson: Be sure the outlet protectors cannot easily be removed by children and are large enough so that children cannot choke on them. It is better to get outlet safety covers that screw into the wall and slide shut when outlets aren't in use. Another way to make unused outlets safe is to place heavy furniture in front of them.

Prevent Strangulation

Think about every item in your home that has a ribbon or string attached to it. Make sure none of those items is near the crib. Don't tie pacifiers, necklaces, toys, or other items around a child's neck.

In fact, don't attach anything with ribbon or string to a child's clothing. When you put the child into his crib, remove a bib or any other clothing that ties around his neck.

Take this admonition a bit further, outside the crib. Drawstrings from the hoods and necks of your child's jackets and sweatshirts can be lethal. (Although in 2011, the CPSC issued a federal regulation for clothing manufacturers prohibiting putting a drawstring in the neck of a child's garment, you still may come across them.) They can catch, not only on a crib, but also on playground equipment. Completely remove any drawstrings from the hood and neck of any child's garment, and if it was purchased new, contact the CSPC to report the article of clothing. (Follow these CPSC recommendations for waist and bottom drawstrings in children's clothing. When the clothing is at its fullest width, the drawstring should not hang out more than 3 inches on each end. There shouldn't be any toggles or other attachments on the drawstring. The drawstring must be stitched into the back so that it cannot be pulled to one side.)

When your child leaves the nursery to go out to the playground, he should not only avoid garments with drawstrings, but he also should not wear oversized clothing, necklaces, or scarves that could get snagged on playground equipment.

According to a new study published in the *Journal of Pediatrics* in 2017, more than 16,800 children under 6 years of age were treated in U.S. emergency departments for window blind related injuries during a 26-year study period. That's almost two per day.

With those statistics in mind, let's take a look at the curtains and blinds you have installed throughout your home. While you may have focused on the color when you dressed windows, there are a few other items to consider once the baby has come to live at home.

Studies have shown that most strangulation deaths from window cords happen when children are in places their parents think are safe: in a crib or child's bedroom, in a playroom or even in the same room with a parent. Where did you place the crib? An infant in a crib near a window can get tangled in a looped window cord running up the slats of blinds or roman shades while playing—or sleeping. Any child wants to look out the window, no matter where her bed may be, and up to the age of 7 she's likely to climb up onto furniture or the window sill to get there. There is a danger she will get caught in a window cord, then fall or jump. Cords cut short can be made long by simply pulling on them. Long cords can spin around the neck of a child in seconds during dramatic play.

The baby monitor won't help here unless it is a video monitor and you happen to be watching it at the time. These deaths are silent. The child won't be able to cry out for help.

Parents for Window Blind Safety (PFWBS), an advocacy group that educates the public on safety and tests window coverings for safety, urges parents and caregivers to use only cordless or cord-restricted window products in their homes. Even if living in a rented residence, parents and others who care for children should replace all window coverings made before 2018 with cordless or cord-restricted products. What to look for:

- Tight Inner Cords. (Loose inner cords that pull out longer than 6 inches are hazardous.)
- Cordless or Cord-Restricted operating cords. Safe window coverings should have no pull cords/chains or have cords/chains that are no longer than 12 inches when pulled, unless covered by a rigid device.

DO IT YOURSELF!

Window Cord Safety Rules
To maximize window cord safety, follow these safety guidelines from Parents for Window Blind Safety:
- Install only cordless window coverings in your home.
- Replace window blinds, corded shades and draperies manufactured before 2018 with cordless or cord restricted products.
- Move cribs, beds, furniture and toys away from windows and window cords, preferably to another wall.
If you have outdated window coverings and cannot replace them:
- Lock cords into position whenever horizontal blinds or shades are lowered, including when they come to rest on a windowsill.
- Make sure inner cord beads are no more than 3 inches below the top of the window covering.
- Cut old operating cords 6 inches from the top of window and tape operating cords to the inside of the headrail or behind slats until new window coverings can be purchased.
- Make sure continuous-loop cords/chains are permanently anchored to the floor or wall. Check often for loose parts.
For more information, go to *www.pfwbs.org*.

(For information about preventing falls from windows, see Chapter 5, "Preventing Falls in the Home.")

Prevent Choking

You may have noticed that infants and toddlers will put anything into their mouths—balloons, small toys . . . small anything! Even food cut into rounds or small pieces can choke a child, as you will see in Chapter 3, "More about the Kitchen: Keeping Your Baby's Food Safe." Putting things in their mouths is one way children explore their world. Choking is a leading cause of unintentional death of children. Children under age 3 are at the greatest risk.

There's another object you may not think comes under the heading of *choking hazard:* the baby bottle. Never prop it up so your baby can "feed herself." Holding your baby during bottle-feeding not only

DO IT YOURSELF?

Making a pacifier . . .
Not!
If you decide to have your baby use a pacifier, don't make one from a bottle top and nipple, or any other such idea Aunt Polly suggests.

Use only a commercially manufactured pacifier from a trusted brand. Look for a one-piece, dishwasher safe variety. (Pacifiers made up of two pieces can pose a choking hazard.) Choose silicone instead of latex because babies can develop a sensitivity or allergy to latex.

affords good bonding, but also reduces the risk of choking, tooth decay, and ear infections.

Another common object that should be inspected is the pacifier. The guard (shield) should be large and firm enough so that it will not fit into the child's mouth, and it should have ventilation holes in case it does. Check the pacifier frequently for holes and tears. And remember what we said about strings: Don't tie the pacifier around the child's neck. (For infants and very young children, no toys should have long strings or cords.)

Teethers, rattles, and squeeze toys should also be large enough that they cannot become lodged in the child's mouth. Inspect such items to make sure they won't come apart, allowing a piece to come loose and be swallowed. Because everything goes in the mouth, a parent must keep everything away from the baby that might possibly find its way into her throat.

Choosing Safe Toys

Any toy you give your child is supposed to be for fun, even if it is also a learning tool. Make sure your child's smile doesn't turn upside down. About 180,000 toy-related injuries are treated in hospital emergency rooms each year. More than a third of those injured are children 5 and under.

Buy Toys Wisely

You don't have to be an expert to carefully choose toys for your infant or toddler. Here are some simple rules to follow.

- Look for quality design and construction.
- Buy toys that are suitable for the age of your child. This is a safety rule that has nothing to do with the child's intelligence. If the label on the toy says *3 years and older,* don't buy it for your 2-year-old. It is likely that these toys have small parts, such as small balls and marbles.
- Read the safety information on the product package. The Child Safety Protection Act prohibits any toy labeled for use by children under age 3 to have any parts that could be ingested or cause choking or aspiration. If you purchase toys from the Internet, be extra cautious. The website may not include product safety warnings, instructions, or age recommendations. In addition, some toys may be manufactured by companies that do not comply with U.S. standards. I recommend that you buy only from vendors you know and trust.
- Don't rely solely on the manufacturer. Even if a toy has no warning label, look it over carefully if your child is under 3. Make sure it poses no choking hazard. Does it have small, detachable parts? Does it have small product accessories? How secure are the eyes, nose, and mouth of that stuffed toy you're considering? Make sure stuffed animals and cloth dolls have well-sewn seams. Does it have loose fur or long hair? You don't want fur, hair, pellets or other stuffing to get into your child's mouth.
- Read the labels on all art materials. The Labeling of Hazardous Art Materials Act requires that all art materials must bear this statement of conformance: *Conforms to ASTM D-4236.* This means the art material has been reviewed by a toxicologist. If any hazardous ingredients have been found, then hazard labeling is required. If the product contains no hazardous materials, there will be no warning, but the statement *Conforms to ASTM D-4236* should still be there.
- Don't buy if you don't see a label. These labels are as follows:
    - For all toys, *ASTM F963.* This label indicates that a toy meets the latest toy safety standards. All toys sold in the U.S. must meet this standard. ASTM F963 includes guidelines and test methods to prevent injuries from choking, sharp edges and other potential hazards.
    - For fabric products, *flame-resistant.*
    - For stuffed cloth toys and dolls, *washable/hygienic material.*
    - For electric toys, *UL.*

- For art materials such as crayons and paint sets, *ASTM D-4236*. (Do not allow children under 12 to use art materials containing cautionary information.)
- Purchase only toys labeled *non-toxic.*
- There is an easy way to identify toys that are too small for your child. If the toy itself or a detachable part fits through an empty toilet paper roll, it is unsafe and should be kept away from children under the age of 3 years and from any child who still puts toys in her mouth. (Keep this in mind when choosing a gift for an older child who has a younger sibling under 3.)
- Never let your child play with plastic bags and packaging material. These items are not toys, and they present suffocation and choking hazards.
- By this time, you are probably wondering what toys *are* okay to buy. For guidance, see Chapter 15, "Debra's Holiday Safety Guide," under "Christmas, Hanukkah, and Kwanzaa."

Whatever toys you buy, check them frequently for broken, ripped, or loose parts. If they cannot be repaired, promptly discard them. Be familiar with the directions and safe use of every toy in your home.

If you're thinking you never knew toys could be so complicated, don't worry. You'll get the hang of it. It really comes down to good sense, once you've become aware of the essential points.

Avoid Potentially Dangerous Toys

When you think about what toys to avoid, the rules are quite practical.

- Avoid toys with sharp edges and points, electrical toys, and toys with heating elements for children under 10 years of age.
- Avoid battery-operated toys. If you do use toys with batteries (a CD player, for example) make sure the battery compartment has a screw closure.
- Avoid propelled toy darts and other projectiles. They can cause cuts or serious eye injuries.
- Avoid toys that are too noisy. No, this isn't to protect Mom's nerves or Dad's ears. Toys that produce loud noises—such as toy caps, noisemaking guns, or high-volume CD players— can produce sounds at noise levels that can injure a child's hearing. (In addition to the loud noise, caps can ignite, causing burns.) Check the noise level before you buy the toy. This applies to squeaky

toys that infants may hold close to their ears. Any loud toy should have directions for safe use—make sure your child follows them.

- Avoid small magnets. High powered magnet sets (like adult desk toys) are dangerous and should not be kept in homes with children. Building and play sets with small magnets should also be kept away from small children. Today's magnets are much more powerful than magnets we used to play with as kids. The serious danger is that the magnet can be swallowed by a child. If more than one magnet is swallowed, they can attract inside the body and cause intestinal perforation, infection or blockage, which can be fatal. (High powered magnets are up to eight times stronger than magnets that are used in toys, warns the CPSC.)

- Avoid button batteries. When swallowed, these coin-size batteries can be deadly. The specific dangers posed by these batteries are covered in Chapter 10, "Common Poisons in the Home."

- Avoid balloons. It may surprise you to learn that balloons lead all other toys in causing childhood death. This concern is not just for babies but for every child under 8 years of age. Certainly you won't allow your toddler to blow up balloons, and you'll want to supervise any play with an inflated balloon. When the balloon bursts, immediately discard deflated and broken balloon pieces. Choose Mylar balloons (shiny, metallic) over latex.

- Avoid fidget spinners. These toys have become extremely popular with people of all ages, including—unfortunately—young children. There are many different kinds of fidget spinners available in stores and online, but all are typically designed with a center bearing and with weights around the perimeter. They are spun in a person's hand. Because a number of incidents have been reported regarding these little toys, the U.S. Consumer Product Safety Commission (CPSC) has issued safety warnings. Spinners of both plastic and metal have small pieces—including batteries—that can be a choking hazard. Fidget spinners should be kept away

---

DO IT YOURSELF!

Keep all toy information in one place.

Keep all information and directions about toys in one drawer or file. This would also be a good place to keep warranty information and serial numbers, in case there is a recall.

Stay up to date on recall information.

(Use a similar system for all your juvenile products.)

from children under three years of age, but children of all ages should be told not to put the toys or small pieces in their mouths and not to play with the fidget spinner near their faces. Choking incidents involving children up to age 14 have been reported.

- Avoid metal jewelry. Not only can such items pose a choking or strangulation hazard, lead and cadmium has been found in inexpensive children's jewelry. In addition, some costume jewelry designed for adults has also been found to contain lead. It is important to make sure children don't handle or mouth any jewelry.
- Avoid small balls. Round objects are more likely to choke children because they completely block a child's airway. Make sure balls, marbles and ball-like objects with which your children play measure more than 1.75 inches in diameter.
- Avoid no-name products and purchase only from reputable retailers. Never buy an item without a manufacturer's name and model number, because it would be impossible to check if the product were recalled.
- Avoid buying older second-hand or used toys; they may contain lead paint.
- Just as you made sure not to hang anything near the baby's crib with a string or ribbon longer than 7 inches, you should continue to avoid toys with strings longer than 7 inches, which can strangle a small child.
- Do not let your baby play with crib toys unsupervised, especially once he begins to push up on his hands and knees.
- In 2008, a law was passed that has made toys and other children's products safer. The Consumer Product Safety Improvement Act included a requirement that toys meet a strong standard and that toys and other children's products be lead free as well as prohibit the use of phthalates—toxic chemicals that were once common in children's toys and child care products. Children's products must be tested by an independent laboratory and be certified that they meet all the applicable regulations.
- If you have a safety issue with any product, including toys and children's products, you can now report it to *SaferProducts.gov,* a database maintained by the US Consumer Product Safety Commission that allows consumers to report safety issues and research a product to see what experiences other consumers have had, even if it has not been recalled.

Everything in the nursery that is meant for the toddler to use should be kept where he can get to it. (See sidebar for guidelines in selecting, building, or remodeling a safe toy box.) If you place your toddler's toys or games in a high place—such as the top of the bookcase—you are inviting him to climb. If you have a shelving unit for toys, keep heavy items on the lowest shelf. Show your child how to put toys away in a safe place, where they won't fall or be tripped over. Don't let your infant or toddler have access to an older child's toys.

Now join the fun. Always supervise your child while he is playing; enjoy this wonderful time.

Safe Practices for Baby's Health

All the rules so far have had to do with objects brought into the nursery. There are also a few cautions about what we and other caregivers do with the baby.

Avoid Flat Spots (Plagiocephaly)

Your baby's skull is soft and his bones are susceptible to pressure. Moreover, if his neck muscles are weak he is likely to turn his head to the same side most or all of the time when he is on his back. This is called

---

DO IT YOURSELF!

Make sure the toy box is safe.
When buying or building a toy box, remember: The best toy box will have smooth, finished edges and have either no lid or a lightweight, removable lid.

If you use a hinged lid, make sure it will stay open in any position and won't close unexpectedly. Inspect it periodically to make sure the support device is still working properly.

If you already own a chest with a hinged, freely falling lid, remove the lid or install a spring-loading lid support. Again, make sure it will stay open in any position and won't close unexpectedly, and inspect it periodically.

Just in case your child climbs inside, make sure the chest has plenty of ventilation holes and the lid does not have a latch.

An easy and safe alternative is to store toys on low-set toy shelves or in plastic baskets (no lids).

a positional preference and can lead to a flat spot on the head. New research seems to be leaning toward very early need for intervention, even at 6 weeks, if your baby has a strong positional preference: either head to the right or head to the left most of the time. If you consult a pediatric Physical Therapist or Occupational Therapist, your baby may avoid a flat spot completely.

To avoid preferential positioning, parents should make use of these positioning options as early as day one at home:

- Alternate the direction your baby's head faces when you place her in the crib.
- Because the baby's natural tendency is to look into the room rather than at a wall, the easiest method of counter-positioning is to change his position in the crib. If you put him down with his head at the head of the crib one time and at the foot of the crib the next, he will turn his head in opposite directions, out into the room.
- If she favors one side or the other in the way she turns her head, regardless of her placement in the crib, move a mobile, toy, or other object of interest (including yourself!) to encourage her to look toward her less favorite direction.
- Alternate the arm you use to hold him while feeding. Support his head at all times so that it is positioned in a straight line and not resting on his shoulder.
- Calm a fussy baby by carrying him in the "football hold," draping his belly over your arm.
- To avoid constant pressure on the back of her head, avoid long periods in car safety seats, strollers and swings.
- One more important thing! Beginning on his first day home from the hospital, play and interact with the baby while he is awake and on the tummy 2 to 3 times each day for a short period of time, 30 seconds to 3 minutes, increasing the amount of time as the baby shows he enjoys the activity. (For a premature or special needs baby, talk to your pediatrician about tummy time play; there may be unique circumstances that need to be considered.) Tummy time is important not only to prevent flat head but also to promote motor development. A good routine to establish is to do tummy time following a diaper change or when the baby wakes up from his nap. Gradually increase the amount of time spent on tummy time play. Always supervise tummy time!

For more tummy time advice, consult your pediatrician and visit the websites in "Helpful Resources" under the tummy time section. Sleep time is not tummy time! Remember: always place your baby on his back to sleep at night and naptime.

Swaddling

The American Academy of Pediatrics (AAP) states there is no evidence to recommend swaddling as a strategy to reduce the risk of SIDS. In fact, according to The Safe to Sleep Campaign of the National Institutes of Health, swaddling can increase the risk of SIDS and other sleep-related causes of infant death if swaddled babies are placed on their stomachs for sleep or if they roll onto their stomachs during sleep. The AAP goes so far as to say there is a high risk of death if a swaddled infant is placed in or rolls to the prone position.

The AAP advises that if you do decide to swaddle, the infant should always be placed on the back. The wrap should be snug around the chest but allow ample room at hips and knees to avoid exacerbation of hip dysplasia. Further, when an infant exhibits signs of attempting to roll, STOP swaddling. There is no evidence with regard to SIDS risk related to leaving the arms in or out during swaddling. According to the AAP, "[d]ecisions about swaddling should be made on an individual basis, depending on the physiologic needs of the infant." (Source: *pediatrics.aappublications.org/content/138/5/e20162938*)

If you choose to swaddle, it's important to discuss the practice and its implications for your child with his pediatrician. Always carefully follow safe swaddling recommendations. For more information about swaddling, visit the American Academy of Pediatrics' website: *www.healthychildren.org*.

Prevent Shaken Baby Syndrome

Another danger for babies is shaken baby syndrome (SBS). No one should shake a baby, not in anger or in play. SBS may be caused by vigorously shaking an infant by the shoulders, arms, or legs. SBS is more likely to occur when an adult is angry, when fun is the farthest thing from anyone's mind. That's why you need your rest!

A baby's neck muscles are too weak to support his head, which is disproportionately large for his body. That's why if he is shaken, his head will flop back and forth, leading to serious injury. In addition, his brain and the blood vessels connecting the skull to the brain are fragile and immature. When a child's head is jerked this way, the brain actually rotates inside the skull cavity, injuring or destroying brain tissue. Blood vessels that feed the brain can also be torn, and when this happens, there is bleeding around the brain. In this circumstance, the blood will pool inside the skull, and that can create even more pressure, lead to further brain damage. Bleeding in the back of the eye (retinal bleeding) is also common in such cases.

A shaken baby can die. Other possible effects range from blindness, spasticity, and seizures to severe motor dysfunction, paralysis, intellectual disabilities, or developmental delays. Children as old as 5 are vulnerable to this type of injury, but babies under 1 year of age are at highest risk.

Whatever the cause, be assured that the baby is not crying to irritate or annoy you. Most of the time you can figure out what the child wants and calm her down by taking care of her immediate needs. After you've tended to the baby's needs, sometimes it is okay to just let her cry. Make sure she's been fed, then check for dirty diapers, and determine the comfort level in the room. After that, put her back into her crib and leave the room. You can still peek in every 10 minutes or so to make sure she's okay, but don't get upset if she continues to cry.

This, too, will pass. It is important to stay calm, because the calmer you are, the calmer your child will be. Sometimes you just have to take a "time-out." Before you lose control, put the baby in her crib and take some time for yourself, away from baby. Some strategies may be helpful here, too; here are some ideas.

- Sit outside the closed nursery door and breathe deeply—a kind of mindful meditation. Breathe in through your nose and out through your mouth. Let the crying fade away; focus on your breathing. (See Appendix G for "Ten Steps to Mindfulness Meditation.")
- Have a trusted adult watch the child while you take a time-out.
- Build a support system among your friends. Meet them regularly at one another's homes or at a restaurant to complain about how tired all of you are or to talk about your babies. It helps to laugh and cry with others who are going through the same things you are.
- Talk to a friend or relative or someone in your support group. Telephone or text, or just talk over the backyard fence.
- Do something you find relaxing: read, exercise, take a bubble bath, play your favorite music. If scrubbing floors or washing windows does it for you, by all means do it!

We've been hearing a lot about mindful meditation lately, and you may believe as a busy parent you don't have time to stop and meditate. On the other hand, a few minutes of time out for yourself and your baby to meditate can help the day go more smoothly. What? A baby meditate? How is that possible? Yes, you and your child can meditate together.

Start with a one-minute daily session with your infant and build up to five minutes as she gets older. A calming sound that focuses you and your baby on a specific noise is one way to do it. Slow everything down for yourself and your child. Don't rush. Just concentrate on the sound. Later you may want to try a game-based technique with activity cards. Such calming activity will stand you and your child in good stead as she grows older.

Make a Wish List

When friends or family ask what baby equipment and supplies you want, be ready with a list. It's a good idea to register at a baby equipment store so you can help gift-givers find what they wish to purchase. This limits the number of items you may have to return or exchange, and there will be fewer hurt feelings. Don't be shy about including higher ticket items, too. There may be a group of people who want to chip in or a grandparent who wants to buy one big gift item. If someone wants to give you a baby shower, say yes! A baby shower is a great way to get everything you need, and it offers a way for friends and family to share in a memorable event—the birth of your child.

Be Thrifty When Buying Baby Clothes

Unlike baby equipment—which I highly recommend purchasing new—children's clothes and cloth diapers can be obtained second hand. I encourage you to take advantage of donations from friends and family. Children grow out of clothes rapidly, so borrowing or swapping makes sense for everyone, and it's good for the environment, to boot! Moreover, clothing resale stores have treasure troves of adorable and practical clothes—often never worn— at half the original price. However, before using any second hand product, including clothes, check with the CPSC to be sure it hasn't been recalled.

Whether or not your child's clothing is bought new or used, carefully examine each piece for safety. Watch out for potential choking and strangulation hazards, such as draw strings, buttons, snaps, ribbons, cords or decorative items. Avoid loosely knitted items, too, because

---

DO IT YOURSELF!

Devise a strategy for calming a crying baby.
No special tools required!
- Hold your baby close to your heart. The sound of your heartbeat is familiar and calming.
- Soothe the baby by lightly rubbing his back.
- Rock him in a rocking chair.
- Sing or hum softly to your baby, or make a steady "shhhh" sound.
- Turn on some quiet music and slow-dance together.
- Take him for a walk outdoors.
- Contact the pediatrician if sickness is suspected.

---

precious fingers or toes could get caught in the thread. Sleepwear for children should be flame resistant and/or tight-fitting (see Chapter 8 for information).

Use Thrift When Buying Diapers, Too

To those of us who try to make decisions with the environment in mind, cloth diapers may seem the best choice. Cloth diapers do not pile up for years in landfills, and they can save you money if you wash them yourself. The choice is not that easy, however, for the environment or for your pocketbook, if cloth diapers are picked up and laundered by a company. The trucks that do the hauling burn gasoline, depleting a resource that is becoming a high demand/short supply commodity.

Although using cloth diapers and washing them yourself can save money in the long run, there is an initial monetary investment. You do have to buy the diapers. Let your family and friends know you plan to use cloth. Hand-me-down diapers are the best! Gently used diapers can be found in thrift stores, too. Cloth diapers have come a long way. New materials and innovative designs make them easier and more efficient to use. To learn more about cloth diapers, go to *www.realdiaperassoctiation .org.*

No matter who washes the diapers, the hot water and energy used to run the washer and dryer also use up a natural resource. Experts disagree about which option is better, but it's likely you'll take the option that fits your lifestyle.

It may be that cloth diapers simply do not fit your schedule or preference. If you choose to use disposables—in conjunction with cloth or all the time—be a frugal shopper. Save money by purchasing generic or store brands, using coupons, taking advantage of sales, shopping at warehouse clubs and buying in bulk. One cautionary note about buying in bulk: your child grows quickly; don't buy so many diapers that he outgrows that size before they are all used.

Review and Safety Checklist

☑ Buy a new crib that meets current safety standards. Look for the Juvenile Products Manufacturers Association certification. Make sure the crib is sturdy, with no loose or missing hardware.

☑ Always lay your baby down to sleep on her back, on a firm, tight-fitting mattress with a crib sheet that fits securely, and remove everything else from her crib.

☑ Never hang anything on or above the crib with a string or ribbon longer than 7 inches. Avoid strings on all infant products, including pacifiers and rattles.

☑ Position any mobile or hanging crib toy out of your child's reach. Remove any hanging crib toys when the baby begins to push up on his hands and knees, or when he is 5 months old, whichever comes first.

☑ Make a safe zone around the crib, bassinet and play yard. Do not position near windows, draperies, cords, hanging wall decorations, heating sources, or climbable furniture.

☑ Buy only toys that are suitable for the age of your child. If a toy fits in an empty toilet paper roll it presents a choking hazard.

☑ Never, ever, shake your baby.

Preventing Injuries in the Kitchen

The kitchen is a favorite gathering place for family and close friends, and your baby will learn quite early that this room is a happy, "happening" place. It is up to the parent to make certain all kitchen happenings are, indeed, happy ones. From the very beginning, you'll need to take precautions in the kitchen with your baby, and the number-one rule is this: Never leave your child unsupervised in the kitchen.

By the way, this may be the first room in which your child will hear the word *no,* so it's a good place to begin teaching her a vocabulary of warning words like *hot, sharp,* and *ouch!*

Keeping Baby Away from Danger
Stay Close and Fasten All Safety Restraints

After placing your child in the high chair, make sure all the straps are buckled, including the crotch strap, and never leave your child unattended in her high chair. Even when you'll be sitting right beside her, be sure to strap her in with the safety harness every time you use the high chair. Don't rely on the feeding tray to restrain or protect her. Without the safety harness holding her securely, she can climb or fall out of the chair or slip between the seat and the tray, possibly getting her head caught and strangling. To prevent a child from slipping down and becoming trapped under the tray, high chairs sold today are equipped with a passive restraint—a crotch post attached to the tray or seat. Even with that safety feature, however, the safety restraint still must be used every time.

Bring Strangulation Prevention into the Kitchen

Remember, too, the precautions taken in the nursery regarding things around the neck. Leave a bib on only while you are feeding your baby, then take it off to avoid a strangulation hazard. Try to buy bibs without strings; bibs with Velcro or snaps are a safer choice.

Set Up a Play Yard

Keep a play yard (also known as a playpen) in the kitchen so your baby can keep you in sight while you prepare food for the family. If you are momentarily distracted, he'll be safe. Get him started in the play yard early by using it instead of the infant seat. Then as months go by, he'll be more likely to play there without protest, even as a curious toddler. This is important, for a toddler can find many ways to get hurt in the kitchen. You can also put the child in his crib or buckle him safely in a high chair in the kitchen. Keep the high chair away from the walls, counters, and table to prevent him from pushing off and tipping the chair over. And be sure to keep all such equipment away from the cooking area!

Keeping Baby Away from What's Hot

Treat the Cooking Area Like a Danger Zone

If range knobs are within reach of your child, take them off when you are not cooking or install stove knob covers or a stove guard. (A little hand can turn the knob, then touch the hot element.) Use only the back burners on your stove for cooking, and keep handles facing the rear so your child cannot grab them, trying to "help." The oven, too, can be a hazard for a small child. I recommend installing an oven-door lock, so the child can't grab the handle and open it while it is hot. An often ignored danger for young children is the oven door itself. Many ovens get hot enough on the outside to cause burns that require hospitalization. The smallest children, those just learning to walk, are the ones most likely to burn themselves on an oven, especially on their hands. Check your oven to see how hot it gets on the outside. Remember: It takes a long time for an oven to cool.

DO IT YOURSELF!

Make your cooking area safe.
• Remove stove knobs when not in use.
• Use only back burners.
• Always wear short, tight-fitting sleeves when cooking: loose clothing can catch on fire.
• Keep pot handles facing to the rear and always use a potholder when reaching for handles.
• Never leave cooking foods unattended—this is the number-one cause of house fires.
• Keep towels, potholders, and curtains away from flames and hot surfaces.
• Clean cooking surfaces regularly to prevent grease buildup, which can ignite.
• Install an oven-door lock.
• Reduce a child's temptation to climb on the range or oven by never storing treats or other tantalizing items above any cooking equipment.
• Maintain a no-baby area around the oven.
• Make sure free-standing ranges and stoves are installed with an anti-tip bracket to prevent the unit from tipping over.

You may have to train older family members and friends along with your baby. He'll hold up his arms to get out of the play yard, and Grandma will take him out, then walk over to show him the food cooking. If she looks away for a moment, his hand or foot can snare something hot, or he can reach out and touch the oven door.

Keep Hot Food and Beverages Away from Edges

Now that you've told Grandma not to bring the baby to the cooking area, she takes him to the kitchen table where she is having her coffee. Um . . . Grandma? Push the coffee away from the edge of the table, out of his reach. If you set him down on the floor, be sure there is no over-hanging tablecloth or mat at the edge of the table. Even with you sitting right there, the baby can reach up, pull the cloth and have hot coffee all over him in a nanosecond. To prevent both of those possibilities, I have two recommendations:

- Invest in spill-resistant mugs to use for hot beverages. Look for a mug that has a spout cover, one that you must actively slide open or press down in order to release the liquid.
- Forego tablecloths and place mats during this period of childhood. (That means less laundry to do—an additional benefit.) All hot foods or beverages, glassware, and utensils should be well away from the edge of kitchen counters or the table.

In addition to taking those precautions, keep children entirely off the floor in the kitchen when anyone is cooking.

Don't Carry Anything Hot While Carrying Your Baby

Even if the hot item is as small as half a cup of coffee, do not carry a child while holding a hot beverage or hot food. Train the rest of the family in this matter, too. You know how a child can wriggle and wiggle. He may choose the exact wrong time to squirm, you'll absently grab for him with the other hand and . . . hot food will be on the baby instantly.

Precautions with the Microwave Oven

There are other ways for a baby to be burned in the kitchen. You know how much it hurts when you sip coffee that's too hot. You don't want that to happen to your child! The greatest danger of offering food that is too hot occurs when it has been heated in the microwave oven. Something may feel cool at the edge but have hot spots in the middle or bottom. That's why I highly recommend that you avoid or use extreme caution while warming up anything in the microwave for your child.

Never Heat a Bottle in the Microwave

A bottle warmed in the microwave heats unevenly and—even after shaking and even though the bottle may feel cool—there can be hot spots in the milk that could burn your baby's mouth and throat. The best way to warm your baby's bottle from the refrigerator is to place it in a bowl of warm water for a few minutes. Then shake and test the temperature by squirting a few drops on your inner wrist. It should feel comfortable—barely warm. Although your baby may seem to prefer it, there really is no health reason to feed her a warmed bottle. In fact, if she becomes accustomed to drinking bottles slightly cold or at room temperature, you'll be saved the time and hassle of heating it and be able to feed her right away, especially when she is crying to be fed.

Avoid Heating Certain Baby Foods in the Microwave

Do not use the microwave to heat baby food containing meats, meat sticks, or eggs. These foods tend to build up hot spots and splatter when the door of the microwave is opened. You or your baby could be seriously burned.

Don't Take Shortcuts

The microwave makes quick work of heating anything, but sometimes you'll be tempted to take an additional shortcut without thinking about the potential danger. This might happen, for example, when you intend to heat commercially prepared baby food the "quickest" way. Never heat solid baby food in the jar it came in. The center will heat to dangerously high temperatures while food in other parts of the jar will stay cool. Before heating, transfer the food to a dish. A 4-ounce dish of solid food cooked on high power will take approximately 15 seconds. Before serving any microwaved food, stir it well with a spoon or fork, then let it stand—30 seconds for that 4-ounce helping of baby food. You cannot tell how hot an item is just by touching the outside of the container, so taste-test the food to see if it's lukewarm, the proper serving temperature. Don't use the same spoon to test the food that will be used to feed your baby. Even your saliva contains bacteria and viruses.

When using the microwave for heating any food, do not use plastic containers. Chemicals used in such plastics could transfer into the food when heated. Avoid this by using only glass or lead-free ceramic cookware approved for microwave ovens.

Don't Let Your Child "Help"

Taking food from the microwave is not an appropriate helping chore for a child. Don't even let her remove coverings or lids from food you have cooked in the microwave—it's dangerous.

Know Your BPAs

BPA (Bisphenol-A) is a chemical component present in polycarbonate plastic; it is used in the manufacture of certain beverage containers and most food can liners. Some research has shown that BPA can seep into

DO IT YOURSELF!

Easy ways to avoid Bisphenol-A and other chemicals
- Use glass and stainless steel baby bottles and containers. (Some manufacturers sell silicone sleeves to prevent glass bottles from breaking.)
- Choose glass, stainless steel or ceramic containers to store food and drinks.
- When buying plastic containers, check the number on the bottom or side. Avoid plastics with recycling #3 (polyvinyl chloride) and #6 (polystyrene foam), and investigate #7 (it can contain BPA). Plastics with the recycling numbers 1, 2, 4, and 5 on the bottom are better choices.
- Use only glass or lead-free ceramic dishware to heat food in the microwave oven.
- Reduce your use of canned foods by using fresh or frozen foods or foods packaged in other containers like glass or cardboard brick cartons.

food or beverages from containers that are made with it. In 2008, the National Toxicology Program of the US Department of Health and Human Services found "clear evidence" that high doses of BPA caused developmental effects in laboratory animals. The agency said at the time that it had "some concern" for effects on the brain, behavior, and prostate gland in fetuses, infants, and children at current levels of exposure to BPA. Four years later, in 2012, the FDA banned the use of BPA in the manufacture of baby bottles and sippy cups, and in 2013, BPA was banned in infant formula packaging.

Most BPA-free plastic products on the market today are actually made with a very similar chemical known as BPS (Bisphenol-S). Recent research reveals it may be just as harmful. Yet another group of chemicals, phthalates, is used to make soft, flexible plastics such as PVC ("vinyl") products and food packaging. Studies find that phthalates may increase allergies and change how male reproductive organs develop.

DO IT YOURSELF!

Protect the baby from harm in the kitchen. Install these items in the kitchen:

- devices that keep cabinet doors locked
- safety latches on drawers
- an appliance lock on your refrigerator, freezer, microwave, trash compacter, and oven

Preventing Injuries Before They Happen

Install Safety Latches

Prevention is the watchword elsewhere in the kitchen, too. Cabinets are awfully enticing to a climbing toddler. Up there is where all the good stuff is kept! No matter how vigilant we try to be, sometimes the little rascal gets a step ahead of us. On the high cabinets as well as those on the floor, install devices that keep the door closed beneath a child's tug but allow it to open easily under the pull an adult can exert. Store knives and other sharp utensils in drawers or cabinets secured with safety latches. Install an appliance lock on your refrigerator, too. Raw meat, as well as medications such as antibiotics, is stored there. One appliance that comes with a lock is the dishwasher. Keep it locked, but just in case, make sure forks and knives are pointed downward.

While you don't want a child under 3 years old to think of a cooking pan as a toy (not knowing the difference when it is full of something hot), some things in the cabinets are not harmful. It won't hurt if the child plays with a wooden spoon and an empty storage container. (Mom and Dad may need earplugs, but that's another matter.) But falling cans can cause a bruise, or worse, and a knife stored on a door or in a drawer can draw blood before you can turn around. There are other dangers lurking behind those cabinet doors as well, such as products that help us keep the kitchen clean or rid the house of insects and other pests. A "poison patrol" will be discussed at length in Chapter 10, "Common Poisons in the Home." Some poisons are look-alikes for good things one eats or drinks, so don't give your toddler a chance to make a fatal mistake.

Stash the Trash

Kitchen trash can contain hazardous objects, as well as spoiled food. Recycling bins also hold potentially hazardous glass and aluminum can lids. Keep the trash and recycling containers securely closed and out of your child's sight and reach.

Keep the Step Stool Inaccessible to Young Children

A step stool is a handy thing to have in the kitchen, but you don't want your child to climb up on it . . . the better to reach something that's dangerous for her to have. When you purchase your step stool, look for one with a handrail that enables you to hold onto it while standing on the top step. Keep it handy for yourself, but not for your child.

Review and Safety Checklist

☑ Don't leave your baby unattended in an infant seat or high chair; buckle up for safety.

☑ Always keep a child away from the cooking area while you are cooking. Keep a play yard in the kitchen for your baby's freedom of movement and your own peace of mind. But remain watchful! Never leave your baby unattended, even in the play yard/playpen.

☑ Remove the range knobs when you are not cooking. Use the back burners whenever possible. Turn pot handles to the back.

☑ Place all hot dishes and beverages, glassware, and utensils in the middle of the table, out of your child's reach. Avoid using place mats and tablecloths.

☑ Don't carry your baby and hot food or beverages at the same time.

☑ Never heat a bottle in the microwave. Before offering microwave-heated food to your child, stir it well, let stand, then taste it to make sure it is only lukewarm.

☑ Use glass or stainless steel baby bottles and sippy cups.

☑ To keep your baby from opening kitchen cabinets, install safety devices or strong rubber bands around knobs.

☑ Securely lock poisonous and hazardous products you keep in the kitchen out of sight and reach of children.

More about the Kitchen: Keeping Your Baby's Food Safe

N ow that you know how to keep your kitchen safe, consider another important thing about the kitchen: food. In the beginning, you'll be breast-feeding or preparing formula. Then you will introduce special baby food (either commercial or homemade) to your child. Later, many foods she eats will be taken from the fare offered to the entire family. When your baby begins to eat solids, she will depend on you to give her food that will not choke her or make her sick.

We'll look at baby food first, then discuss tap-water safety, which is quite important when you are using water to prepare formula or food for your baby. After that we'll discuss practices for avoiding food-borne illness.

Baby Food Basics

Keeping your baby's food safe is an important part of keeping the baby herself safe. From the time you prepare or purchase a food product until you store it and eventually feed it to your little darling, you will want to take great care.

Pay Attention to the Package

The first precaution you'll take is at the store. Check the *use by* date on any product your baby will ingest; if the date has passed, don't buy it. Check again when you remove baby food, juice, or formula from your cabinet to give to your baby. If the expiration date has passed, don't use it. Wash the lid before opening, then listen for the pop. If the lid of the baby food jar doesn't pop, it has not been sealed safely, so don't use it. After opening, check for chipped glass or rusty lids. If you see any such defect, do not use the product.

Learn What and How to Feed Your Baby to Encourage Good Health

Ask your pediatrician for any feeding guidelines you should follow specifically for your baby, and inquire about any possible need to use bottled water or sterilized water when mixing formula. No matter how or what you feed him, always wash your hands thoroughly before beginning food or formula preparation. There are other general guidelines for feeding him:

- When preparing baby formula, carefully follow the manufacturer's recommendations. The American Academy of Pediatrics recommends for the first year of life a baby should drink breast milk (breast is best) or iron-fortified formula. Cow's milk shouldn't be added to the diet until your infant is a year old. Cow's milk doesn't provide the proper nutrients for your baby. If you give cow's milk to your child between 1 and 2 years of age, it should be whole milk. (Note: the AAP says your child's doctor may recommend reduced-fat (2%) or low-fat (1%) milk if your child is obese or overweight, or if there is a family history of high cholesterol or heart disease. Always check with your child's pediatrician before switching from whole to reduced-fat milk.) Breastfeeding can continue after 12 months of age, for as long as is desired by mother and baby.
- Most babies are ready to start solid foods at around 6 months. Here are the developmental signs that indicate your baby is ready. Baby can: sit up unsupported; has good control of his head and neck; shows interest in food when others are eating; opens his mouth wide when offered food on a spoon; turns his face away to let you know he is full or just not hungry; uses his lips to remove food from the spoon; is able to keep some food in his mouth.

Thoroughly discuss starting your baby on solid foods with your baby's pediatrician.

- Use caution when warming up food or beverages for your baby. Set the bottle of formula, expressed breast milk, or other liquid into a bowl of warm water for a few minutes. Do not use the microwave (see the section "Precautions with the Microwave Oven" in Chapter 2 for a more thorough discussion). You can bypass heating the bottle altogether. It is perfectly all right to give your baby her bottle chilled or at room temperature. In addition, you should not use the microwave to heat meats, meat sticks, eggs, or jars of food. Hot spots created in the microwave can burn your baby's mouth.

- Test before feeding. Always shake the bottle and test the temperature by dropping some of the beverage on your inner wrist. After stirring food thoroughly, test it by tasting it to see if it's lukewarm. Remember: don't use the testing spoon to feed your baby; your saliva contains bacteria and viruses that could harm your child.

- Unless you know for sure all the food will be eaten in the first sitting, do not feed your baby directly from the jar. Put a small amount in a clean bowl and feed your child from that bowl. After feeding, discard any leftovers remaining in the bowl, jar, or bottle. Just as your saliva contains bacteria that might harm your baby, bacteria from the baby's saliva can grow and multiply; neither refrigerating nor reheating will prevent or destroy the contaminants.

- Be sure containers are clean. Prior to first use, sterilize new bottles, nipples, and rings. After each use, clean reusable bottles, caps, nipples, and other utensils by washing them in a dishwasher or in hot tap water with dishwashing liquid; rinse in hot water. If your water is from a well or is not chlorinated, you should sterilize utensils before use.

Store Baby Food Safely

Store unopened baby food and formula in a dry, cool area. Read the label to see if there are special storage recommendations. Leftovers may be refrigerated or frozen. Once opened, baby food (solids or liquids) should not be left at room temperature for more than an hour. (The guideline for food safety is usually 2 hours, but with infant food—for safety's sake—many experts recommend reducing that time to 1 hour.) When you store food or liquids that have been opened, don't trust your memory. Label the container with the date the product was originally opened.

Freezing unused prepared formula is not recommended, but it can be refrigerated. Use within 24 hours. Don't let it stand in an open container; keep it covered. Store unused baby food in the original jar with a tightly closed lid. To know whether a particular product can be frozen, you will read the manufacturer's recommendation on the label, of course, but there are some general guidelines for time limits for refrigerating or freezing baby food products:

- *Strained fruits and vegetables:* refrigerate for 2 to 3 days, freeze for 6 to 8 months
- *Strained meats and eggs:* refrigerate for 1 day, freeze for 1 to 2 months
- *Meat/vegetable combinations:* refrigerate for 1 to 2 days, freeze for 1 to 2 months
- *Homemade baby foods:* refrigerate for 1 to 2 days, freeze for 1 month. (Making your baby food is convenient and economical, and you'll have more control over the variety and texture. You'll also want to take care of the milk you hand express or pump as carefully as you handle other baby food. For information on the proper handling and storage of human milk, go to *http:// www.cdc.gov/breastfeeding/recommendations/handling_breast milk.htm.*)

Tap Water Safety

Infants drink more fluids per pound of body weight than anyone else in the family, so parents are right to be concerned about the safety of their tap water. This worry is particularly apt because the immature system of an infant makes the baby especially vulnerable to microbial contaminants sometimes found in tap water.

In general, there is no need for alarm in the United States, due largely to the Safe Drinking Water Act of 1974 and its amendments (passed in 1986 and 1996). As a consequence of the Act, the EPA has issued primary drinking water standards called Maximum Contaminant Levels for about 90 contaminants. These standards limit the amount of each substance allowed to be present in drinking water. United States public water suppliers are required to perform water-quality monitoring to ensure that the water remains free from unsafe levels of contamination. Utilities must notify customers when tests show the water does not meet EPA standards.

The EPA has also issued secondary drinking water standards concerning the taste, odor, color, and certain other aesthetic qualities of drinking water that, although they may be undesirable, are not considered to pose a health risk. The EPA recommends these guidelines as reasonable goals, but states are not legally required to comply. However, some states have adopted their own enforceable regulations.

You can be more at risk for contaminants in your water if it comes from a private water supply or from a smaller water system that may not have enough monetary resources to hire trained specialists or make necessary improvements. Private water supplies are defined as domestic systems serving homes supplied by on site individual wells. These private domestic water supplies are not regulated under the Safe Drinking Water Act. Individual homeowners in these situations must take steps on their own to test and treat their water as necessary, to safeguard against any possible serious health effects. Therefore if you receive your drinking water from a private well, you should have your water tested periodically.

Learn about Contaminants Sometimes Found in Drinking Water

If you receive your drinking water from a public water system, your water supplier must notify you by newspaper, mail, radio, TV, or hand-delivery if your water does not meet EPA or state standards or if there is a waterborne disease emergency. The notice will describe any precautions you need to take. In addition, it's also very important to read your water supplier's most current Drinking Water Consumer Confidence Report (also known as a Water Quality Report).

It is no overstatement to affix the label enemy to such water quality parameters as bacteria, parasites, nitrates, trihalomethanes, arsenic, chromium-6, radon, lead, and pesticides that may be lurking in your water. Any of them can potentially harm your baby.

Microbial Pathogens (Bacteria and Parasites)

These contaminants (cryptosporidia and giardia, for example) are common in lakes and rivers contaminated with human and animal fecal waste. They can cause diarrhea, nausea, and stomach cramps, and they are most dangerous for infants, the elderly, and immune-compromised adults. Pregnant women should take precautions as well. (The coliform bacteria E.coli is the test indicator for fecal contamination that indicates other pathogenic bacteria and viruses are likely present. There should be zero coliform bacteria in drinking water.)

Nitrates

A high nitrate level is likely to be found in rural areas where ground and surface water is contaminated with animal waste or runoff from nitrogen-based fertilizer. Infants are most at risk because nitrates reacting with the hemoglobin in the baby's blood produce an anemic condition known as *blue baby*. Left untreated, the condition can be fatal. Unless you know your water is safe, do not drink the water if you are pregnant. And don't give your baby any nitrate-contaminated water or food, or formula that contains nitrate-contaminated water. Boiling does not help. In fact, prolonged boiling of water contaminated by this element increases the nitrate concentration. Either buy bottled water from a quality source or invest in a home treatment device.

Important Note: Do not feed home-prepared spinach, beets, turnips, carrots, or collard greens to a baby younger than 6 months of age. These home-prepared vegetables may contain large amounts of nitrates.

Trihalomethanes (THMs)

When chlorine—the chemical used to disinfect water— combines with naturally occurring organic matter like decaying leaves, THMs are formed. THMs have been linked to bladder and rectal cancer. The current federal level for THMs is 80 ppb. Because one can also inhale THMs, reduce your shower time and have good ventilation in your bathroom.

Chromium-6

Also called hexavalent chromium, chromium-6 is the chemical best known for its role in the Erin Brockovich story. This toxin can leach into water either naturally or from industrial runoff. While the EPA classifies chromium-6 as a known carcinogen, to date, there is no federal standard on the maximum allowable amount of chromium-6. The EPA has set a regulation for total chromium, but that includes chromium-3, which is a naturally occurring chemical and essential human nutrient.

Arsenic

This contaminant has been linked to cancer, skin lesions, endocrine disruption, and nerve damage. The Maximum Contaminant Level for arsenic in drinking water is 10 ppb. Water systems must meet this standard.

Test for Other Toxic Contaminants

Radon, lead, and pesticides can also contaminate drinking water. For a thorough discussion of specific risks associated with these elements and the best ways to test and treat for them, please refer to Chapter 11, "Environmental Hazards."

Radon, a radioactive gas, can seep into ground water, and your family can be exposed to it not only through drinking water, but also by showering or washing dishes. However, indoor air pollution by radon is usually more of a health concern.

For a thorough discussion about lead, please refer to the section "Lead" in Chapter 11, "Environmental Hazards."

Pesticides (including herbicides, insecticides, and fungicides) pose more risk for families living in active farming communities.

Investigate Your Water Supply

If you are served by a public water system, contact your local water utility. You'll find the phone number on your water bill. Ask the following three questions:

1. Where does my drinking water come from?
2. How is this water treated?
3. What contaminants are tested?

Then read a copy of the utility's most current Drinking Water Contaminant Analysis Report. The law requires all community water systems to furnish this information to you in an annual Consumer Confidence Report by July 1 for the previous calendar year. This report may also be available on the website of your water utility. Or look up your city's water in the Environmental Working Group's national tap water database, *www.ewg.org/tapwater.*

Take particular note of any violations.

Also call your local Health Department and Department of Environmental Protection to ask what contaminants they test for and request copies of their analysis reports. The reports cannot tell you what happens to your water between the treatment plant and your tap. You will need to have your own water tested for lead and copper. If your water has a blue-green tinge or if your fixtures are stained blue-green, you should suspect high copper levels.

If you suspect illness, or see, taste or smell changes to your drinking water, ask your utility to visit your home and test the water.

Heed the Safety Guidelines If You Are on a Private Water System

Call your state and local health departments or your local cooperative extension agent. Ask about groundwater problems in your area and inquire about past, present, or potential problems. Ask about testing. Some local health departments test water for free; some do so for a fee. You can also contact your state laboratory certification office for a listing of certified drinking water laboratories in your state. The EPA recommends annual testing for nitrates, total dissolved solids and coliform bacteria, which, though generally harmless, may indicate other contamination. If a problem is suspected, you may need to test more frequently and for more potential contaminants. Well water should also be tested for lead. Testing for lead is particularly important if you have lead pipes, soldered copper joints, or brass parts in the pump.

Additional testing is indicated if any of these conditions or activities is present or nearby: intensive agriculture, a dump, a landfill, a factory, a gasoline service station, auto repair shop, or a dry-cleaning operation. Ask your local health department and your cooperative extension agent for guidance on what specific contaminants should be tested for.

Test Your Water

You should have your water tested by a state-certified laboratory. To get the names of certified labs nearest you, call your state laboratory certification office or, if you prefer, call the EPA Safe Drinking Water Hotline: (800) 426-4791.

To be on the safe side, do not have your water tested by a company trying to sell you a water treatment device. If the results from their lab indicate you do have a serious problem, get a second opinion from a different lab before spending money on an expensive water treatment product.

Find the Right Water Treatment for Your Family

Do your homework! There is a wide range of prices; don't buy more than you need. If a $20 pitcher will do the job necessary to protect the tap water in your home, why buy an under-the-sink unit that costs $1,000?

To find a quality product and one that is certified to remove the specific contaminants found in your drinking water, you can choose among the following independent, non-profit organizations:

- NSF International. (877) 867-3435; *www.nsf.org.*
- The Underwriters Laboratories, Inc. (888) 547-8851; *www.ul.com /water.*
- The Water Quality Association. (630) 505-0160. *www.wqa.org.*

Both NSF International and Underwriters Laboratories, Inc., test and certify home water treatment units. The Water Quality Association classifies units according to the contaminants they remove as well as listing units that have earned their "Gold Seal" approval. Water treatment units certified by these organizations will indicate certification on their packaging or labels.

Follow the Manufacturer's Instructions for Maintenance or Get a Maintenance Contract

Any product requires periodic maintenance or replacement. The unit that insures the purity of your water is no exception. In fact, a filter that is poorly maintained can be worse for your health than drinking the water without the filter. A dirty filter can be a breeding ground for bacteria, and it can cause contaminants to begin flowing back into the water.

Knowing yourself is important. Can you—and will you—follow instructions for proper maintenance? If you are not so inclined, it is best to purchase a contract from the dealer.

Comparison-Shop If Bottled Water Is Your Choice

The FDA regulates bottled water as a food. It generally imposes quality standards equivalent to the EPA's drinking water standards. Treat bottled water as you do foods; refrigerate after opening. Whether bottled water is any safer than the water from your tap can be disputed. In fact, some bottled water is simply repackaged municipal water. The source of the water and the practices of the company selling it can cause quality to vary. Contact the manufacturer of your favorite brand, ask how they treat their water, and request a copy of their most recent water analysis. The International Bottled Water Association represents the bottled water industry. You can contact them by calling (800) WATER-11 or by visiting their website, *www.bottledwater.org.* NSF International and

Underwriters Laboratories, Inc. also provide testing and certification of bottled water.

Consider using a water filter to purify tap water instead of buying bottled water. Not only is bottled water expensive, but it also generates large amounts of container waste. You can bring along your own reusable glass or stainless steel water bottle when traveling or at work.

Drinking bottled water or using an in-house treatment system is a temporary solution. The underlying problem remains. Actively support efforts to upgrade the supply and treatment of safe drinking water and to protect water supplies from industrial and agricultural pollution. And do your part at home by composting, recycling, and properly disposing of hazardous material.

Foods That Can Choke

Young children are particularly at risk for choking because of their poor chewing and swallowing abilities and narrow airways. Always consider the size, shape, and texture of any food before giving it to your baby, and consult your pediatrician for specific guidelines for foods appropriate for your child's feeding stage. The American Academy of Pediatrics (AAP) recommends that children younger than 4 years should not be fed any round, firm food unless it is chopped completely. Trust yourself. If you have any doubt about whether a food is safe for your child, don't serve it. Even with all the precautions considered below, a piece of food may lodge in a child's throat. This point cannot be made too often: Take an infant/child CPR and first aid course.

Know What Not to Serve

The AAP lists the highest risk foods, advising that children under 4 years of age should not be given any of these: hot dogs or sausage; hard, gooey or sticky candy; peanuts, nuts, and seeds; whole grapes; chunks of meat or cheese; marshmallows; chunks of peanut butter; popcorn; chunks of raw fruits or vegetables (such as carrots or apples); chewing gum.

Among the candies you should avoid giving to your child are jelly beans, lollipops, fruit roll ups, and gummy bears. (Oh, no! You'll have to watch what Uncle Charlie is hiding in his pocket.) Other foods that can choke your child are pretzels, chips, berries, raw cherries with pits, cherry and grape tomatoes, celery, string beans, raw peas, and dried fruits. Any sticky food can cause your child to choke. Never spoon-feed peanut butter to your child. If you do serve it, put a thin layer of it on a cracker or sandwich (but not on soft white bread), and always serve it with a beverage.

Use Caution Away From Home

When you take your baby to a restaurant, be alert from the moment you walk in. At the table, be especially alert if adult munchies—freebies like peanuts and popcorn—are part of the fare. These should be kept out of your baby's reach. Even food you've ordered may cause a toddler to choke, especially if he's so hungry he shovels the food into his mouth. Before he gets his hands on it, cut the food into bite-size pieces, and if he's within reach of your plate, cut up your food, too. On the way out of the restaurant or any other business where impulse items are displayed at the checkout station, watch your baby's hands. He can grab hard candy or any other small item and have it in his mouth before you notice.

When you travel with your child in a car, avoid feeding him in the car. An unexpected bump or swerve could make him choke. If the driver is the only adult in the car, it may be impossible to attend to the child quickly.

Teach Table Manners for Safety

Good manners at the table make eating safer. Teach your child to sit upright, eat slowly, take small bites, and chew each bite thoroughly. Always supervise your child's mealtime to make sure she understands and follows the rules. Eating should always take place while sitting. Walking, running, or playing should not accompany eating; neither should talking, laughing, or giggling. Eating is not a multitasking endeavor. Enjoying a meal is good for the digestion and disposition, but fun at the cost of safety is a no-no.

Start early with being careful about how your baby eats. An infant should never have his bottle propped up. Hold your baby during bottle feeding. Hold the baby in a semi-upright position and angle the bottle accordingly. I mentioned this in Chapter 1, but it bears repeating. Not only is this a special bonding, snuggle time, it also lessens the risk of choking. Drinking from a propped bottle can lead to tooth decay and ear infections, as well. So don't prop!

Many choking accidents happen when an older sibling feeds her younger brother or sister. Be sure your older children understand why you follow these rules.

DO IT YOURSELF!

Prepare food so it won't choke your child.
• Grind, grate, chop, or mash and moisten food.
• Cook or steam vegetables and firm fruits to soften them.
• Remove all bones from fish, chicken, and meat before cooking.
• Cook food until it is soft enough to easily pierce with a fork.
• Remove pits, skin, and seeds from all fruits and vegetables.
• Cut round foods lengthwise into thin strips. (Any round or cylindrical object can fit snugly in the windpipe.)
• Remove the skin of grapes, and cut the grapes lengthwise and into quarters.
• If you choose to serve a hot dog, remove the peel and slice the hot dog into quarters lengthwise; then cut it into small, bite-sized pieces. (Opt for the nitrate-free varieties.)
• Cut food into small pieces, no larger than ¼ inch, or thin strips that can be easily chewed.

What You Need to Know about Food-Borne Illness

Americans used to think food-borne illness was a problem found only in other parts of the world, but recent headlines have told a different story. In fact, according to the Centers for Disease Control and Prevention, 48 million Americans get sick and 3,000 die from food-borne illnesses each year. Infants and children are more at risk because they have less-developed immune systems. Common symptoms include diarrhea, abdominal cramping, fever, blood, or pus in the stool, headache, vomiting, and severe exhaustion. In a child, these symptoms must be treated immediately because such illness can be life-threatening.

Be aware that symptoms may appear as early as half an hour after the contaminated food is consumed, or they may not develop for several days or weeks. When trying to nail down the cause of symptoms, don't just look back over 1 or 2 days.

Know What Foods to Avoid

Some foods are more likely than others to be contaminated with harmful bacteria. Children, pregnant women, people with weakened immune systems, and older adults should avoid the following foods:

- *Soft, unprocessed cheeses.* Soft cheese made from unpasteurized milk—such as feta, Camembert, blue-veined cheeses, Panela, queso blanco, and queso fresco—can harbor bacteria of the genus Listeria. (Note: They're okay to eat if the label says "Made with Pasteurized Milk.") In babies it can cause a brain infection that can lead to brain damage; in pregnant women it can cause miscarriages and stillbirths. (For more information about Listeria, go to *www.cdc.gov/listeria.*)
- *Raw (unpasteurized) milk and foods made from unpasteurized milk.*
- *Raw or undercooked eggs or products made with raw or undercooked eggs.* Egg dishes should be cooked to a temperature of 160°F or by a visual check, with both the yolk and white firm, not runny. Hard-cooked eggs should be safe for everyone in the family to eat. Do not give your children soft-cooked or runny eggs. Don't use recipes in which eggs remain raw or only partially cooked, such as homemade ice cream, mayonnaise, Caesar salad dressing, or French toast.
- *Don't eat cookie dough either.* (I can hear you groaning.) We're talking about the homemade batter that's made with raw eggs, which can be contaminated with Salmonella. My words of wisdom: Eat your homemade cookies cooked. However, if you simply cannot give up raw cookie dough or if you prefer eating undercooked eggs (sunnyside up, over easy or soft-boiled), consider using pasteurized eggs. These eggs can be found in most supermarkets and are labeled "Pasteurized."
- *Raw or undercooked meat, poultry, fish, and shellfish.* Foods from animals, such as meat, poultry, fish, and shellfish, when eaten raw or undercooked, can contain life-threatening bacteria and viruses. Children, pregnant women, people with weakened immune systems, and older adults should not eat raw fish or shellfish such as oysters, shrimp, crab, clams, sushi, or sashimi. Nor should they eat meat or seafood ordered undercooked, such as rare hamburger, beef, lamb, pork, or fish. Always use a food thermometer to be sure foods are safely cooked. (See the temperature chart on a following page.) Do not eat hot dogs, luncheon meats or deli meats unless they are reheated until steaming hot.
- *Raw sprouts, such as alfalfa, clover, or radish.* These have been associated with Salmonella and *E. coli* 0157:H7. Cook sprouts thoroughly to kill off the bacteria.

- *Unpasteurized juice or cider.* These can contain bacteria, including *E. coli* 0157:H7 and Salmonella. Pasteurization is a heat process that destroys harmful levels of bacteria in liquids. Pasteurized products include shelf-stable items unrefrigerated in the grocery store, such as those packaged in cans, bottles, and juice boxes. Warning: Some fresh juices and ciders—commonly sold at roadside stands, country fairs, and juice bars, as well as those kept on ice or in refrigerated display cases at grocery stores—are unpasteurized. Always check for labeling information on juice packages. When in doubt, ask. If you have purchased a product and are unsure whether it has been pasteurized, bring it to a boil for a minute, then cool before drinking it or giving it to your child to drink.

Take Care with Fruits and Vegetables

As we have seen in recent headlines, fruits and vegetables can harbor disease-causing bacteria. How can this happen? The answer lies at a number of points along the route the food takes to get to your table from the field: a) fertilization with raw manure, b) irrigation with contaminated water, c) rinsing the plants with contaminated water, and d) contamination by food handlers. Before offering any raw produce to your family, it should be thoroughly washed under clean running water, which has an abrasive effect. This is true even for organic fruits and vegetables. As an extra measure of caution, wash pre-washed labeled products, too. If appropriate, use a small scrub brush. It's important to wash the skin and rind, too, even if it will not be eaten. This prevents pathogens from being transferred from the rind or skin to the inside of the fruit or vegetable when it is cut. When you're washing lettuce and other leafy vegetables, discard the outer leaves. Separate the inner leaves and wash thoroughly. Take extra care, because such leaves are harder to clean thoroughly.

You don't have to buy expensive veggie cleaners, although they are available in stores. Instead, use a vinegar and water solution. Don't use dishwashing liquid to wash produce; it is difficult to avoid leaving residue, and most soaps are not meant to be consumed.

Know When to Avoid Mushrooms and Honey

Wild Mushrooms

Some common species of wild mushrooms are capable of causing poisoning or even death. Only an expert with specialized training can distinguish the edible kinds from the others. Eat only mushrooms you've purchased in the grocery store or the ones you've raised at home from cultures bought from reputable sources.

Honey

Do not serve honey to children under age 1. It may surprise you to learn that honey should never be given to a baby. This food—healthful for most of us—may contain bacterial spores that can cause infant botulism, a rare but serious disease that affects the nervous system of young babies. Don't add honey to your baby's food, water, or formula, and don't dip your baby's pacifier in honey.

Follow Guidelines for Safe Food Handling

Shop Carefully

- Go to reputable stores that are clean and well maintained and that have meat and poultry supplied by USDA-inspected or state-inspected plants. Fish should be purchased at markets where supplies are bought from state-approved sources.
- Carefully consider what you put in your shopping cart. Do not purchase foods beyond the *sell by* or *use by* dates.
- Do not choose foods with torn or broken packaging. Do not buy cans or glass jars with dents, cracks, or bulging lids— this can be a sign that the food contains harmful microorganisms.
- Buy only meat, poultry, or seafood that has been refrigerated or frozen. Place these foods in plastic bags to keep juices from leaking out.
- Look for grade A or AA refrigerated eggs with clean, uncracked shells.
- Select fruits and vegetables that are free of mold and decay. Make sure the produce isn't brownish, slimy, dried-out, or damaged.

Store Food the Right Way

- Choose perishable foods last—right before grocery check-out— then go straight home and refrigerate or freeze the food immediately. If you have other errands, do them before shopping for perishable food or pack a cooler with ice packs for your perishable food.
- Use an appliance thermometer to be sure the refrigerator is 40°F or below and that the freezer is 0°F or below to keep food at safe temperatures.

- Store canned goods in a cool, dry place. Never put them above the stove, under the sink, in a damp garage or basement, or anywhere else exposed to high or low temperature extremes. Store cans of high acid foods such as tomatoes and other fruit up to 18 months; store cans of low acid foods such as meat and vegetables 2 to 5 years.
- Most fruits and vegetables should be stored in the refrigerator to avoid spoilage. However, some produce should be stored only at room temperature in a clean, dry, well-ventilated place away from direct sunlight. These are: garlic, onions, potatoes and sweet potatoes. Don't put them under the sink, because leakage from pipes can damage food.
- Other produce that should be stored at room temperature until ripe, then put into the refrigerator, are apricots, avocados, bananas (skin will darken but the actual fruit is unaffected), mangos, melons, nectarines, papaya, peaches, pears, plums and tomatoes. (Do not put vegetables in a crisper section with fruits; keep them separate to prevent exposing vegetables from ethylene gas naturally produced by some fruits.)
- To speed ripening, place produce in a loosely closed brown paper bag or ripening bowl. Plastic bags may slow ripening, but they may also increase spoiling.

Thaw with Safety in Mind

Do not thaw food on the counter! Bacteria multiply quickly at room temperature. The following are safe options.

- Defrost food in the refrigerator. This requires planning ahead because several hours or days are required.
- Put the food in a watertight plastic bag and immerse in cold water; change the water every 30 minutes.
- Use the microwave. Follow the manufacturer's directions for your microwave model. Foods defrosted by this method should be cooked right away.
- Keep in mind that foods defrosted in cold water or in the microwave should be cooked right away.

Keep Everything Clean When Preparing Food

Wash your hands with soap and warm water for at least 20 seconds— and use a nail brush— before and after handling food or food utensils.

HAND WASHING 101

- Wet your hands with clean (warm or cold), running water. Turn off the tap.
- Apply a mild liquid soap or clean bar soap. Do not use antibacterial soap.
- Rub your hands together vigorously until a soapy lather appears. Continue for at least 20 seconds. (Hint: It takes about 20 seconds to sing the alphabet song.)
- Scrub under the fingernails, between fingers, and around the tops and palms of the hands.
- Rinse thoroughly under clean, running water.
- Dry hands with a clean towel or air dry them.

Teach your toddler how to wash his hands. Make it fun by singing a song (such as the alphabet song). To add some silliness, make up your own words while you wash your hands together.

Note: In September 2016 the FDA banned over-the-counter/consumer antibacterial soaps containing certain active ingredients, stating there is no evidence that antibacterial soaps are any more effective than plain soap and water at preventing the spread of germs. In fact, the use of antibacterial soap may contribute to antibiotic resistance. The CDC supports the FDA's decision and does not recommend the use of antibacterial soaps over regular soap for the general public (not including healthcare professionals).

Clean the counters, tables, cutting boards, and utensils thoroughly with hot, soapy water after use and before using them on another food. Wash the lids of canned foods and drinks before opening to keep dirt from getting into the food. Clean the blade of the can opener frequently. Even if you're trying to save the planet by limiting the use of throwaway products, I highly recommend that you consider using paper towels to clean up all kitchen surfaces, especially those touched by raw meat, poultry, or seafood juices. Harmful bacteria multiply quickly on kitchen towels, sponges, and cloths. If you choose to use cloth items, wash them often in the hot water cycle of your washing machine. If you choose to use sponges, discard them often.

Cook Food Thoroughly

Always use a food thermometer to be sure foods are safely cooked. Thermometers are inexpensive and easy to use; just follow the instructions and make sure you have the right kind for the job you're doing. Don't think you can tell by looking whether meat is safely cooked. Your child's hamburger must be cooked to an internal temperature of at least 160°F. It is important to always use a thermometer because hamburgers can turn prematurely brown before reaching a safe temperature. When reheating leftovers, heat to 165°F. Ready-to-eat food such as hot dogs, luncheon meats and deli meats should be heated until they are steaming hot or 165°F. Here's a safe minimum temperature chart from the USDA.

(For more information, go to *www.fsis.usda.gov/wps/portal/fsis /topics/food-safety-education/get-answers/food-safety-fact-sheets/safe-food -handling/safe-minimum-internal-temperature-chart/ct_index.*)

PRODUCT	MINIMUM INTERNAL TEMPERATURE AND REST TIME
Beef, Pork, Veal & Lamb Steaks, chops, roasts	145 °F (62.8 °C) and allow to rest for at least 3 minutes
Ground meats	160 °F (71.1 °C)
Ham, fresh or smoked (uncooked)	145 °F (62.8 °C) and allow to rest for at least 3 minutes
Fully Cooked Ham (to reheat)	Reheat cooked hams packaged in USDA-inspected plants to 140 °F (60 °C) and all others to 165 °F (73.9 °C).
All Poultry (breasts, whole bird, legs, thighs, and wings, ground poultry, and stuffing)	165 °F (73.9 °C)
Eggs	160 °F (71.1 °C)
Fish & Shellfish	145 °F (62.8 °C)
Leftovers	165 °F (73.9 °C)
Casseroles	165 °F (73.9 °C)

Serve and Handle Food Carefully

- *Perishable foods.* Never leave perishable food at room temperature for more than 2 hours (one hour if the temperature is 90ºF or higher). This includes raw and cooked meat, poultry, and seafood products. Once fruits and vegetables are cut, it is safest to also limit their time at room temperature. If perishable food is left at room temperature for more than 2 hours, bacteria can grow to harmful levels.
- *Leftovers.* When refrigerating, divide the leftovers into shallow, covered containers so the food will chill rapidly and evenly.
- Know when you should not cook. If you have an infected sore or cut or have been sick with vomiting or diarrhea, do not prepare or handle food. The germs that are making you sick can easily be passed to your family, and your baby is the most at risk.

Reduce the Risk of Pesticides in Your Child's Diet

Our children may be exposed to pesticides from residues found in their food. Although pesticides are discussed in greater detail in Chapter 11, "Environmental Hazards," I'll quickly mention here some ways you can reduce the risk of pesticide residues in your child's diet.

When Possible, Go Organic

You may choose to purchase foods and beverages that are certified as organically grown and processed. Organic food is produced according to certifiable guidelines, using renewable resources and conserving soil and water. For animal products, *organic* means antibiotics and growth hormones are restricted. For fruits, vegetables, and grains, restrictions pertain for most conventional pesticides, petroleum- or sewage-sludge-based fertilizers, bioengineering, and ionizing radiation.

Before a product can be labeled *organic,* a government-approved certifier inspects the farm where the food is grown to make sure the farmer is following all the rules necessary to meet USDA organic standards. Companies that handle or process organic food must be certified as well. Today, many groceries carry organic food, but you can also grow your own chemical-free produce in your backyard. When you grow your own, you have more control over your food. This can be a great family activity.

WHEN TO WASH HANDS

Before . . .
- preparing bottles or feeding children
- giving or applying medication to child or self
- preparing food
- eating
- treating a cut or wound.

After . . .
- preparing food
- eating
- using the bathroom
- assisting child in using toilet
- changing diapers (wash baby's hands, too!)
- blowing one's nose
- covering a sneeze
- wiping child's runny nose
- cleaning up spit, vomit, or similar substances
- handling pets, pet cages, or other pet objects
- handling animal waste
- engaging in outdoor activities
- handling trash
- cleaning the house
- working or gardening outdoors
- removing gloves used for any purpose
- treating a cut or wound.

Other times . . .
- when hands are visibly dirty
- when someone in the house is sick, wash hands more often

Lower Pesticide Risk in Other Foods

- Choose a variety of foods. This will give your family a better mix of nutrients and reduce the likelihood of exposure to a single pesticide.
- Trim the fat from meat and poultry. Pesticides tend to accumulate in the fatty tissues of animals.
- Remove the skin from chicken and fish.
- Discard the fat in broths and pan drippings.
- Wash produce under clean running water, which has an abrasive effect. Follow the guidelines described in the topic "Take Care with Fruits and Vegetables," earlier in this chapter.
- Peel skin or outer leaves.
- Buy produce in season. Not only is it less expensive, but it is also less likely to have been treated with fungicides and other preservatives.
- Buy from local growers. In this way you avoid buying food shipped over long distances or stored over long periods of time and there is accountability for the manner in which it was produced. It also provides tremendous support to the local farmers. Moreover, it can often mean lower prices, too. I think local produce is fresher and better tasting than anything in the grocery store. To help find family farms, farmers markets, and other sources of sustainable produce grown in your area, go to *www.localharvest.org.*

Buying organic can be more expensive, so you may have to make hard choices. It's most important to buy organic when you purchase fruits and veggies that, if not grown organically, have the highest pesticide residues. Every year, The Environmental Working Group (EWG) releases its annual Shopper's Guide to Pesticides in Produce. The guide lists "The Dirty Dozen"—the conventional fruits and veggies that have the most pesticides, and "The Clean Fifteen"—the ones that have the fewest. For detailed information about the produce on both lists, go to *www.ewg.org/foodnews/list.php.*

Choose Fish Wisely: Limit Exposure to Mercury

Fish and shellfish can be important parts of a healthy and balanced diet. They are good sources of high quality protein and other essential nutrients. They are also a major source of omega-3 fatty acids. Not all fish have the same amount of omega-3s; sardines and salmon are some of the best options. However, some fish contain mercury at levels that can be harmful to a young child or unborn baby.

About half of the mercury in the environment comes from natural sources such as volcanoes, while human activity accounts for the other half. Whether from natural or man-made sources (such as coal-burning or other industrial pollution) mercury can be converted by bacteria to its most dangerous form—methylmercury— which accumulates in the fatty tissues of fish and other animals. While trace amounts of mercury are present in most types of fish, it becomes most concentrated in large, predatory fish such as swordfish and sharks. Most harmful to the developing brains of unborn children and young children, mercury can affect cognitive, motor, and sensory functions. Mercury can also impair the immune system and can damage DNA.

In 2017 the U.S. Food and Drug Administration (FDA and the Environmental Protection Agency (EPA) issued revised new guidelines regarding fish consumption for pregnant women or women who may become pregnant, as well as breastfeeding mothers and parents of young children. See chart below. Discuss these recommendations with your health care provider.

Advice About Eating Fish

What Pregnant Women & Parents Should Know

Fish and other protein-rich foods have nutrients that can help your child's growth and development.

For women of childbearing age (about 16-49 years old), especially pregnant and breastfeeding women, and for parents and caregivers of young children.

- Eat 2 to 3 servings of fish a week from the "Best Choices" list OR 1 serving from the "Good Choices" list.
- Eat a variety of fish.
- Serve 1 to 2 servings of fish a week to children, starting at age 2.
- If you eat fish caught by family or friends, check for fish advisories. If there is no advisory, eat only one serving and no other fish that week.*

Use this chart!

You can use this chart to help you choose which fish to eat, and how often to eat them, based on their mercury levels. The "Best Choices" have the lowest levels of mercury.

What is a serving?

To find out, use the palm of your hand!   For an adult 4 ounces   For children, ages 4 to 7 2 ounces

Best Choices EAT 2 TO 3 SERVINGS A WEEK			OR	Good Choices EAT 1 SERVING A WEEK		
Anchovy	Herring	Scallop		Bluefish	Monkfish	Tilefish (Atlantic Ocean)
Atlantic croaker	Lobster, American and spiny	Shad		Buffalofish	Rockfish	Tuna, albacore/ white tuna, canned and fresh/frozen
Atlantic mackerel		Shrimp		Carp	Sablefish	
Black sea bass	Mullet	Skate		Chilean sea bass/ Patagonian toothfish	Sheepshead	
Butterfish	Oyster	Smelt			Snapper	Tuna, yellowfin
Catfish	Pacific chub mackerel	Sole		Grouper	Spanish mackerel	Weakfish/seatrout
Clam	Perch, freshwater and ocean	Squid		Halibut	Striped bass (ocean)	White croaker/ Pacific croaker
Cod		Tilapia		Mahi mahi/ dolphinfish		
Crab	Pickerel	Trout, freshwater				
Crawfish	Plaice	Tuna, canned light (includes skipjack)		**Choices to Avoid** HIGHEST MERCURY LEVELS		
Flounder	Pollock	Whitefish				
Haddock	Salmon	Whiting		King mackerel	Shark	Tilefish (Gulf of Mexico)
Hake	Sardine			Marlin	Swordfish	Tuna, bigeye
				Orange roughy		

*Some fish caught by family and friends, such as larger carp, catfish, trout and perch, are more likely to have fish advisories due to mercury or other contaminants. State advisories will tell you how often you can safely eat those fish.

www.FDA.gov/fishadvice
www.EPA.gov/fishadvice

For further guidance on which fish are richest in healthy omega-3 fatty acids, lowest in mercury contamination and sustainably produced, use the Environmental Working Group's (EWG) Seafood Calculator to get your custom seafood list, based on your age, weight and more. Go to *www.ewg.org/research/ewg-s-consumer-guide-seafood/seafood-calculator.*

Take Steps to Reduce Arsenic in the Diet

Based on the FDA's findings with respect to inorganic arsenic in rice, the agency offers the following advice to parents and caregivers of infants. It is consistent with advice given by the American Academy of Pediatrics.

- Feed your baby iron-fortified cereals to be sure he is receiving enough of this important nutrient.
- Rice cereal fortified with iron is a good source of nutrients for your baby, but it shouldn't be the only source, and does not need to be the first source. Other fortified infant cereals include oat, barley and multigrain. (When introducing any new foods, the AAP recommends doing so slowly and watching for any reactions.)
- For toddlers, provide a well-balanced diet, which includes a variety of grains.

Also based on the FDA's findings, it would be prudent for pregnant women to consume a variety of foods, including varied grains (such as wheat, oats, and barley), for good nutrition.

Published studies, including new research by the FDA, indicate that cooking rice in excess water (from 6 to 10 parts water to one part rice), and draining the excess water, can reduce from 40 to 60 percent of the inorganic arsenic content, depending on the type of rice, although this method may also remove some key nutrients.

(Note: The AAP also recommends limited intake of all sweet beverages, including juice. Infants are encouraged to eat whole fruits that are mashed or pureed. Fruit juice offers no nutritional benefits for infants younger than 1 year. Toddlers and young children are encouraged to eat whole fruits instead of drinking juice.)

(Sources: *www.fda.gov/ForConsumers/ConsumerUpdates/ucm493677 .htm; www.healthychildren.org/English/ages-stages/baby/feeding-nutrition /Pages/reduce-arsenic.aspx; pediatrics.aappublications.org/content/139/6/ e20170967)*

Please consult your child's pediatrician and your healthcare provider for more information.

(See the sidebar "Prepare food so it won't choke your child" and the section on arsenic under "Tap Water Safety" earlier in this chapter.)

Review and Safety Checklist

☑ Choose a clean, well-maintained grocery store when shopping for your family. Check food packaging—whether you're buying baby food or food for the rest of the family— and check it again when you are ready to serve it. Heed *sell by* and *use by* dates. Avoid foods whose packaging contains dents, chips, and rust.

☑ Know when and when not to use the microwave to heat your baby's food.

☑ Don't store opened baby food too long; label unused food when you put it in the refrigerator.

☑ Investigate your water supply. If you are on a public water system, read a copy of the latest Consumer Confidence Report. If you are on a private water system, contact the state and local health departments or a cooperative extension agent for recommendations. Take appropriate steps to ensure safe consumption by filtering tap water, or avoiding it entirely by buying bottled water.

☑ Keep firm, round foods away from your child, and take care with sticky foods. Stay equally vigilant when you take your child to a restaurant.

☑ To reduce the risk of food-borne illness, avoid:

☑ soft, unprocessed cheeses

☑ raw, runny, or soft-cooked eggs

☑ raw or undercooked meat, poultry, fish, or shellfish

☑ raw sprouts

☑ and unpasteurized milk, juice, or cider.

☑ Children, women who are planning to become pregnant, and pregnant or nursing women should not eat fish that is high in mercury.

☑ Thoroughly wash fruits and vegetables before using. Toss out damaged produce.

☑ Take care with wild mushrooms and never give honey to a child in the first year of life.

☑ Buy only meat, poultry, or seafood that has been refrigerated or frozen. Place these foods in plastic bags to keep juices from leaking out.

☑ Refrigerate perishables.

☑ When cutting boards, utensils, plates, counters, and hands have been touched by raw meat, poultry, or seafood, wash them thoroughly before they come in contact with cooked food or raw vegetables and fruits.

☑ Wash lids of canned foods and beverages before opening, clean the can opener frequently, and use paper towels to clean kitchen surfaces.

☑ Choose a safe thawing method that suits you and your family, either in the refrigerator, in a sealed bag in cold water, or in the microwave oven.

☑ Always use a food thermometer when you cook.

☑ Before eating, insist on clean hands all around, from baby to the one who serves the food.

Bathroom Safety

In the olden days (that were not so golden), folks had to go outside to use the privy, and the greatest danger—aside from the risk of falling in—was the possibility of running into a skunk or stepping in what the chickens had left behind. Those dangers were rendered obsolete with the advent of the modern, indoor bathroom, and since that time we've come a long, long way. However, even if you have the most luxurious bathroom with the most up-to-date accoutrements, there may be worse dangers there than our great-great grandparents could have imagined. Never assume your child is too young or has motor skills too poorly developed to get himself into trouble. He may have talents of which you are unaware. You may think your docile child would not have the desire to climb up onto counters or open cabinets, but he is an explorer, discovering a new world. Take measures to keep your child away from danger.

A hook-and-eye latch high on the outside of the bathroom door will enable you to keep your toddler out of the bathroom, even if you have been distracted for a moment or two. When you have read more of this chapter, you'll better understand why this is a good idea. On the other hand, a locked door can become a problem if the lock is engaged inside the room—and your toddler is inside alone. (In fact, she may have been the one who locked the door!) If your bedroom or bathroom door has an inside lock, practice opening it from the outside against the day when you'll need to do it in a hurry. Some locks are relatively simple to open with a small screwdriver. You can also remove the door locks, but a less drastic action is to place a towel over the tops of doors to prevent them from closing completely.

DO IT YOURSELF!

Making the doorstop safe.

When is a doorstop a hazard? When your child can reach it. The spring action will catch her attention, and she can pull off the plastic tip easily, presenting a choking hazard. There are two solutions:

• Replace the stops near the floor with ones near the top of the door.

• Install solid one-piece doorstops made of polyethylene. These are available in hardware stores and through mail order catalogues.

Measures to Prevent Burns

Any family member can receive a serious burn from scalding water coming from the faucet of a sink, bathtub or shower. Children are particularly vulnerable because they have thin skin. The risks of severe scalding can occur with temperatures over 120°F. In fact, according to Safe Kids Worldwide, an average of twelve children ages 14 and under die from scald burn-related injuries each year. Children ages 4 and under account for nearly all of these deaths. Water at a temperature of 140°F will produce third-degree burns on a child in 3 seconds! A temperature 20 degrees lower gives you about 5 minutes to react before such a burn can occur, and it will still get both your clothes and your dishes clean.

Stay Out of Too-Hot Water!

The first measure in protecting the family, therefore, is to make sure your water heater is set so it cannot scald your child. (See the sidebar for steps you can take and devices you can buy.)

Be Vigilant Around Hot Water

With or without devices, there are precautions for saving your child from being scalded.

• When filling the bathtub, start with cold water, then add hot. Turn off the hot water first. This way you reduce the likelihood that the water will get too hot or your child will get burned from the hot metal faucet.

• Before letting your child get into the water, move your hand back and forth for several seconds, testing its feel on your skin and making sure there are no hot spots. Before your child enters the tub, be sure the faucet is completely turned off.

• When placing your child in the tub, position her with her back facing the faucet. If she doesn't see the faucet, she won't be tempted to play with it.

- To avoid the danger of your child bumping her head, as well as touching hot metal, you may wish to purchase a foam-rubber protective device that slips over the faucet and handles.
- Bath mats or non-slip strips put directly on the bottom of the tub should always be used to keep your child from slipping and falling.

Around Any Water: Be There!

Carefully and constantly supervise! Regardless of the number of devices you install and the care you take in making sure the temperature is safe, there is no substitute for being there. Always be there! Constant, undistracted adult supervision is essential when a young child takes a bath or shower.

Never Leave Your Child Alone with Any Water

Never leave, even for a moment, for although the temperature is just right and the baby's bottom is firmly in place on a bath mat, there is still a danger of drowning. I highly recommend not using a bath seat. Parents get a false sense of security from such items and may be tempted to leave the baby unattended for a moment. These products

---

DO IT YOURSELF!

Prevent scalding.
- Set the thermostat for your water heater at 120°F or lower.
- If you live in an apartment building, check with the property manager to make sure the water heater is set to this temperature.
- Test the water coming out of the tap again, after you have made adjustments.
- Be aware that 120°F water can still burn your little one, so always mix hot water with cold water before it touches your child's skin.
- For additional protection, you can purchase an antiscald device. Install it on the tub faucet or other bathroom fixtures. This device shuts off the water before it reaches a temperature that could harm your child.
- You can also buy a thermometer to make sure the temperature is safe. A comfortable water temperature for the child is near his own body temperature, around 98°F-100°F. Never exceed a water temperature of 100°F.

BATH TIME SAFETY CHECKLIST

- Use a non-slip bath mat or non-slip strips in the bottom of the tub.
- NEVER run the water with the child in the bathtub.
- Fill the tub with just an inch or two of water.
- Test the temperature of water before putting your child in the tub. A water temperature of 98°–100°F is recommended.
- Before bathing your baby, have within arm's reach all the necessary supplies, i.e., wash cloth, mild soap, baby shampoo, 2 soft towels, fresh diaper and outfit.
- NEVER leave a baby unattended for a second, even with older children. If you need to leave the bathroom, take baby along. Empty bath water immediately after use.
- ALWAYS keep one hand on your baby at all times.
- When taking your own bath, remember to never leave a tub with water unattended, even when your toddler is sleeping. Note: Tub baths can begin any time after the umbilical cord falls off and the circumcision site is completely healed. You should give your baby sponge baths before this occurs.

are intended as bathing aids—not safety devices—and they will not prevent drowning if the child is left unattended. In fact, these products have been linked to numerous deaths. The baby can climb or fall out of the seat, or the seat can tip over. When this happens, the baby can slip down under the seat and be held under water. (Instead of a bath seat, consider using a small, plastic bathtub. See section below.) If the doorbell or phone rings while your child is in the bathtub, either ignore the sound or take your child with you to the phone or door. Immediately empty the water out of the tub or any container after you have used it.

Drowning is the leading cause of injury death for children ages 1 to 4, and the second leading cause of injury death among children ages 1 to 14, according to the CDC.

Children ages 1 to 4 most often drown in swimming pools, hot tubs, and spas. Children under age 1 most often drown in bathtubs, buckets, and toilets. Standing water anywhere poses a drowning hazard. In fact, a small child can drown in as little as 1 inch of water. A toilet, bucket, or pail may be as dangerous as a pool or ocean. Keep small children away from any liquid-filled bucket; particularly hazardous are 5-gallon buckets. Because a child's head is so heavy, he cannot push himself out if he topples into water headfirst. A momentary lapse of adult supervision, even a few seconds—the time it takes to answer the phone or door—can cause tragedy. Drowning is a silent death; it is unlikely that a child with his nose and mouth in the water will be able to scream.

Take these precautions: Empty any bucket or container immediately after you have finished using it, and store it out of reach. It's especially important for pails and buckets kept outside to be turned upside down because they can collect rainwater. If you are temporarily interrupted while using a bucket, move it to a safe place. Keep the toilet seat cover closed at all times when it is not in use and install a toilet lock. This device is easy for adults to unlock, but it will keep your child out. Make the bathroom off-limits except for bath and potty times.

Choose Safe Bath Equipment

Select an infant or child's tub made of sturdy plastic that safely supports your child. Use a contoured design to help raise your infant when he can't sit up on his own. The bathtub should have slip-resistant backing to keep it from sliding. Do not choose a tub with rough edges that can scratch your baby. If the plastic infant or child's tub is used in a regular bathtub, make sure the drain is open so excess water doesn't fill the larger tub's reserve.

Purchase an infant bath tub that was manufactured on or after October 2, 2017. Such bath tubs are required to meet the new CPSC safety standards, having improved warning labels and stronger locking mechanisms. And always follow the Bath Time Safety Checklist.

Care with Electrical Appliances

Don't you feel better knowing how easy it is to avoid these dangers? Because you exercise caution, bathroom water will neither scald nor drown your baby. Now look around the bathroom. No matter its size, there may be other dangers lurking there.

Remember That Water and Electricity Do Not Mix

Do you have appliances with electric cords in the bathroom? Chances are, you have a hair dryer or curling iron, and possibly an electric razor that must be plugged in. Water and electricity don't mix. If an electrical appliance gets wet when it is plugged in, the user can be electrocuted.

Certainly, if such an appliance is dropped into water, the person in the water—especially a child—can be killed.

Have a Professional Install Ground Fault Circuit Interrupters

When purchasing any electrical appliance, look for the mark of a recognized testing lab, such as UL (Underwriters Laboratories), CSA (Canadian Standards Association), or ETL (Electrical Testing Laboratories). Unless you live in an old home, you probably have GFCIs (ground fault circuit interrupters) installed. Here's the time frame: The National Electrical Code has required GFCIs in outdoor receptacles since 1973, bathroom receptacles since 1975, garage outlets since 1978, and receptacles in crawl spaces and unfinished basements since 1990. If you do not have them installed in those places in your house or you need to take temporary measures, you may purchase portable GFCIs at a hardware store for plugging into electrical outlets. If you do not already have them, you'll do better in the long run to have a qualified electrician install GFCIs in all electrical receptacles inside and outside your home near water sources. (This is not a place to cut corners.) The GFCI automatically shuts off electricity flow when it detects electricity entering a body and grounding the flow. Even with GFCIs in your bathroom, avoid using an electrical appliance there or around other water sources. If the worst happens—perhaps at the home of friends— and an appliance does fall into the water, do not pull it from the water until you are certain it is unplugged. Always keep electrical cords out of the reach of your children.

Always Unplug an Appliance Immediately after You Use It

Even if the switch is off, the appliance is still electrically live if it is plugged in. Since the early 1990s, hair dryers have had built-in shock protection devices to prevent electrocution if they fall into water. Use a dryer with a large, rectangular plug. Store such appliances safely out of the reach of your child, preferably outside the bathroom. Never place or store any appliance where it can fall or be pulled into the bath or sink, and watch out for the cords! A dangling cord is a mighty temptation to a child. An appliance falling on his head may not electrocute him, but he can certainly be injured by it.

Don't Leave a Hot Appliance Unattended

All the approval ratings and safety devices in the world won't keep that appliance from getting hot. Don't forget that it will stay hot for at least

5 minutes after being turned off. To avoid skin burns, put it down on a stable surface so that it won't fall, and don't leave it unattended while it's still hot. Store it after it has cooled. One appliance designed to be hot is a bathroom heater, but don't use it without a guard around the heating element. Even with the guard, do not leave a functioning heater and a child alone together in a room.

Poisons in the Cabinet

We've taken steps to protect the child from being scalded, drowned, and electrocuted, but there is one more grave danger in this necessary room. Think about it. What do you keep in the cabinet under the sink or in the so-called medicine cabinet?

Find the Poison and Lock It Up

Now is the time to move poisonous products you kept safely in the bathroom before you had a child. These include mouthwash, prescription medicine, iron supplements, and over-the-counter medicine such as pain relievers. Any of those products can be mistaken by the child for something he has been allowed to have. (See Chapter 10, "Common Poisons in the Home.") Securely lock poisonous and hazardous products (such as razors, tweezers, and scissors) out of the sight and reach of children.

Safe Disposal of Unused Medications

It used to be easy. Just flush. But scientists tell us this is not a good alternative in most cases. Putting medications down the drain can contaminate the water supply, not only affecting our drinking water, but also causing harm to fish and wildlife.

As you go through your medicine cabinet for safety's sake, throwing away medications you no longer use, do not flush them or pour them down the sink unless those particular medicines have a notice on the label and are listed on the FDA website (FDA.gov) as appropriate for flushing. Such medicines are especially dangerous if accidentally ingested by children or pets, and they have specific disposal instructions for flushing down the sink or toilet as soon as they are no longer needed, when they cannot be disposed of through a medicine take-back program. The take-back program is the first and best option. To find a medication disposal program in your area, call the Poison Help Line, 1-800-222-1222, or visit *www.disposemymeds.org.* You can also get information about safe disposal from local law enforcement agencies. If your old medications are not on the flush list at FDA.gov, and there is no take-back program near you, the FDA recommends:

1. Mix medicines (do not crush tablets or capsules) with an unpalatable substance such as dirt, kitty litter, or used coffee grounds.
2. Place the mixture in a container such as a sealed plastic bag.
3. Throw the container in your household trash or take to a hazardous waste dump. (Garbage cans should be kept securely covered and placed out of reach of children.)
4. Scratch out all personal information on the prescription label of your empty pill bottle or empty medicine packaging to make it unreadable, then dispose of the container.

Review and Safety Checklist

Protect your child from scalding in the tub or at the sink by:
- ☑ Adjusting your home water heater thermostat to 120°F or lower
- ☑ Turning on cold water first, then adding hot, when filling the bath tub; turn off the hot water first
- ☑ Feeling the water for hot spots and mixing it around before the child gets into the tub
- ☑ Using a thermometer to see that the water temperature is 98°F to100°F

Protect your child from being electrocuted or burned by:
- ☑ Having ground fault circuit interrupters installed in the bathroom and anywhere a receptacle and a water source are present
- ☑ Making sure your appliances have the *UL, CSA,* or *ETL* mark of approval
- ☑ Keeping electrical appliances away from sinks and tubs, unplugging appliances after use, and tying up electrical cords so they don't dangle
- ☑ Putting hot appliances on a stable surface after using, away from small hands
- ☑ Carefully supervising the use of any appliance that gets hot and promptly putting it away after it cools

Protect your child from drowning by:
- ☑ Staying with your child every second he is in the bathroom, especially in the tub

DO IT YOURSELF!

Practice safety with medicine.
- Never call medicine candy, even if you are trying to get the child to take the medicine.
- Don't take your medicine in front of your child; she'll try to imitate you.
- Don't let her play with medicine bottles.
- Never give medication in the dark and be sure to put your glasses on. You may pick up the wrong medicine or give an inaccurate dosage.
- Keep all your medications in their original, child-resistant packaging, but remember that these lids are child-resistant, not childproof. They buy you only some extra seconds.
- Securely close caps after using a medication and promptly return the item to its place after using it, locked away, out of sight and reach of children.
- Properly dispose of unused medications. Do NOT flush unused medications or pour them down a sink unless the label says to flush them. If possible, return your unwanted medicine to a take-back program. Don't put pills in your handbag, or in pockets, where a child can easily get them.

☑ Installing locks on the toilet and always keeping the lid closed
☑ Immediately emptying the water from the tub, sink, or any container after it has been used
☑ Keeping your child away from any liquid-filled bucket or container

Protect your child from poisoning by:
☑ Locking up poisons that are commonly kept in the bathroom
☑ Securely closing the child-resistant cap after using a medication and promptly returning the item to its proper place

Part II

Safety Measures
for Every
Living Space

B efore a child came to live in your home, you could afford to be
careless about where you put things. Your only problem then was
whether you'd be able to find your handbag or your keys, or an earring
or watch. It's best to start creating new habits for yourself early, even
before your baby is born. Once she arrives, you'll have plenty to do.

Not only will you want to change the pattern of tossing small items
on a convenient chair, low table, or shelf, but you will also— before
your baby begins to crawl—want to get into the habit of regularly
and carefully inspecting your home for small objects. Crawling around
every room is one way to do it if your knees will take the pain. Look

under beds, furniture, and cushions, and in bags and pockets that a child might be able to reach.

To understand what you're looking for, go back to the axiom from Chapter 1: Children put everything in their mouths. Look for anything that is small enough to fit: coins, small batteries, small balls, marbles, crayon pieces, keys, jewelry, paper clips, buttons, pop-can tops, plastic bags, wrappers, nails, tacks, screws, safety pins, and removable rubber tips on doorstops.

Also look for items on your child's clothing that might come off. Use Velcro instead of buttons and avoid jeweled decorations that the child can pull off. If your baby's clothes or toys have plastic labels or decals, remove and properly discard them before he pulls them off himself . . . and puts them in his mouth.

With that introduction to "all-through-the-house" caution, let's move to some specific hazards in the home. In Chapter 5 you'll learn how to prevent two kinds of fall-related injuries: first, the child's falling from stairs, windows, or furniture, and second, heavy items that can fall on the child. Chapter 6 takes us to areas outside the house, as well as the garage, workshop, and basement. For the backyard, we will discuss safety guidelines for pools and around the playground and barbecue grill. Safety with pets is the topic in Chapter 7. We detail fire safety in Chapter 8 and gun safety in Chapter 9.

Dangers surrounding common poisons we keep at home are considered in Chapter 10, and Chapter 11 provides guidelines concerning environmental hazards that can affect the entire family but especially babies.

Special problem areas that are part of having an office at home are explained in Chapter 12, with a note about knowing your own limitations. Even if your office is at home, there will still be times when you'll need to hire a sitter or find a reputable child care center. You'll learn how to do it wisely in Chapter 13. To finish the section, Chapter 14 lists items that should be part of your first aid and disaster supplies kits.

Preventing Falls in the Home

Falls are a leading cause of hospitalization and emergency room visits for children. Someone might joke that we need not worry about small children falling because they don't have as far to fall, but every conscientious parent knows infants and toddlers are more vulnerable to serious injuries caused by falls. If you must leave your baby alone for a moment, make sure she is in a safe place, such as a crib. If she is on a changing table, a bed, or any furniture from which she can roll over and fall off, do not leave her for a second.

The greater risk for infants is associated with falls on stairs and from furniture. For toddlers, falls from windows present the greater risk. On the other side of the coin is the danger of being a victim of something falling. In addition to discussing things that are not designed to fall but do, I'll consider a product that is supposed to fall: the garage door. The issue is not to keep the door from falling, but to make sure there is nothing or no one under it when it comes down. Just in case, an auto-reverse device equipped with an entrapment protection feature is crucial.

Stairs
Keep Stairways Lit and Clear of Clutter
One of the simplest ways to make stairs safe is to light them. This helps everyone in the family, but it is especially important if you have a baby in your arms. Have a light switch at both the bottom and the top of the

DO IT YOURSELF!

What to do with plastic bags . . .
- Tie plastic bags and wraps in knots and discard, or store them locked away from children.
- Don't forget to remove all dry-cleaning bags from your closets. A child can suffocate when a plastic bag covers his face.

stairs. Keep battery-backup night-lights at each end, as well, in case of power failure.

In fact, no part of the house should be dark when your family is moving about. Power-failure night-lights are like regular night-lights except that they automatically switch on as emergency lights any time the power fails. Prices start at around $10 each. In addition to placing them at each end of the stairs, put them in halls, bedrooms, and bathrooms, too, so that the entire family will always have a lighted path.

Night-lights at floor level, especially those that look like toys, may attract your crawling baby to the socket. If possible, install a night-light in a socket out of the baby's reach. Use night lights with child-safety features; look for ones that completely enclose the bulbs and have safety tabs that hinder a child's ability to remove it from an outlet.

Even when stairs are well lit, anyone can trip on objects left there. Stairs and landings should be kept free of any clutter. If you are in the habit of placing items on the stairs to be picked up the next time you go up or down, break the habit. And don't allow toys, boxes, or books to be placed there at any time of the day. Steps are not storage units. Another tip: Don't wax the stairs or the landing area.

Purchase and Install Safety Gates, and Know When to Take Them Down

When your baby begins to move—even before he can crawl— install safety gates at the top and bottom of stairs, carefully following the manufacturer's instructions. Hardware-mounted gates should be installed at the top and bottom of the stairs. A pressure gate, which attaches to the walls with pressure rather than with screws, is suitable for less hazardous locations such as for separating rooms on the same floor and in hallways. Never put a pressure gate at the top of the stairs; such a gate can give way if a child leans on it. Make sure the gate at the top of stairs swings only one way: away from the stairs.

When your child is old enough to climb over a gate or has learned to open it (when she is about 2 years of age), remove it. When it comes down to it, a gate should be difficult to climb over, no matter what the child's age. Choose gates with vertical slats rather than horizontal ones, and make sure the slats are no more than 2 3/8 inches apart. Even better, choose a gate made from fine mesh or Plexiglas. Never use older accordion-style baby gates because they pose an entrapment and strangulation hazard. These gates have V-shaped openings along the top edge and diamond-shaped openings between the slats that are large enough to entrap a child's head.

No matter what materials are in the gate or how it is attached, do not rely on the gate (or any other baby equipment) to keep your precious one safe. A gate should never be used as a substitute for close adult supervision. Once your child is moving around on her own, with or without gates, the size of the space between stair railings is important. The space should never be more than 3 1/2 inches wide. (See the sidebar under the section in this chapter titled "Balconies, Decks, and Porches.")

Teach Safe Walking

Practice walking up and down the stairs with your toddler. Teach him that he should always hold on to the hand railing when going up or down. (Be sure there is a sturdy railing on both sides that your child can reach.) Don't be shy about inventing solutions of your own. When my children were first starting to climb steps, I positioned the bottom gate on the third or fourth carpeted step to allow them some supervised climbing experience on the bottom few stairs. That way a fall would not be from a great height. No matter what kind of surface—rugs, tile, or wood—is in your home, don't allow children to play on the stairs.

Keep in mind that children (and adults, too!) can easily slip on scatter rugs. If possible, to prevent tumbles, remove the rugs or secure them with double-faced adhesive carpet tape or nonskid matting under each rug.

Furniture

Look around your home. Nearly every item can either fall or be fallen from. The possibility of falling furniture may be a novel idea to you if you're new at this parent-of-a-toddler business, but there are a variety of ways furniture can tip. Your tiny beloved may fall against the furniture, causing it to tilt, or he may climb up on it, perhaps in an innocent effort to retrieve something he wants. Down will come baby, bookcase and all! Maybe he'll try to move the furniture, or perhaps he simply wants to sit on it. It's possible that he's just trying to be helpful by opening or closing a door, drawer, or compartment. If it's moveable, it can fall.

If you're used to making your own improvements around your home, you can probably figure out some of the precautions you should take to keep furniture from falling. To enable you to cover all the bases, I have a few hints.

On average, a child dies every ten days from a TV or furniture tip-over incident, according to CPSC data from 2011 to 2013. Properly mounting or anchoring a TV, dresser and other large furniture can prevent these tragic incidents.

Avoid Buying Certain Items

Don't purchase furniture items with wide shelves or footholds; such pieces can encourage climbing. Avoid freestanding items, such as floor lamps and standing coat racks (which are sometimes as free-falling as they are freestanding). Choose storage furniture (bookcases, cabinets, TV stands and dressers) with wide and deep, stable bases that sit directly on the floor and have a low center of gravity.

Securely Anchor to the Wall All Large and Top-Heavy Furnishings

Heavy items such as bookshelves, heavy appliances (including the kitchen oven), and entertainment centers can tip even when they are set against a wall. Use brackets, braces, or wall straps—they are lost-cost!—and look for furniture that is sold with anti-tip devices. Install them right away. Use the same preventive measures for cabinets, dressers, chests, and bureaus, too, but with furniture like this, you must go one step further. If it has drawers, install child-resistant locking devices to prevent children from opening the drawers and using them to climb up. Even if your chest or bureau is secured to the wall, a child climbing on the drawers could slip and suffer a deadly fall. Avoid placing tempting items—such as toys or the remote control—on top of furniture or TV.

Important Note: In 2016, IKEA recalled 29 million MALM and other models of chests and dressers. To date, very few of these dressers have been accounted for. Eight children died in tip-over accidents. Parents are urged to stop using any recalled IKEA dressers.

Televisions

With bigger screens and smaller backs, flat-screen TVs create a greater tipping hazard. Always follow the manufacturer's instructions to ensure that you have a secure fit. Mounting flat-screen TVs to the wall is the preferred method to prevent them from toppling off stands. Televisions that are not wall mounted should still be anchored to the wall. When anchoring the TV to a wall, using the proper anchoring kit designed for your TV is essential, and it is important to screw the anchors into the studs in the wall. If you are mounting your big screen to a low piece of furniture, use the furniture straps or angle braces that are specified by the TV manufacturer. These are usually included with the TV or the TV stand that is sized to accommodate your new TV. Do not, under any circumstances, set the braces or straps aside for possible use later.

Older and bulky TVs (CRT TV) are more tip prone, too, because they are heavier in the front. When they fall, the heavy TVs can fall with the force of up to 12,000 pounds. Be sure to place such a TV on a low, wide base—on furniture designed to hold a television—and push it as far back as possible. Check to make sure the size and weight limit of the stand will hold your TV, and still anchor it to the wall or the TV stand. Shelves, nightstands and dressers are not made to support TVs, especially when the drawers are opened.

The CPSC recommends recycling older, unused TVs, as they are a potential deadly danger. Learn how to recycle at *greenergadgets.com*.

Arrange Furniture with Safety in Mind

Table lamps are safer at the back of a table, close to the wall. For lighting rooms where a toddler roams, a ceiling light fixture or wall lamp is best. To keep the center of gravity low, place heavy items on lower shelves. Anything heavy and able to be tipped should be stored in an inaccessible place. In fact, any knickknacks or breakable items should be kept out of your

DO IT YOURSELF!

Another use for duct tape!

You don't have to buy corner covers. Instead, use padding and duct tape. Put the padding over the top and sides of the corner and use duct tape to affix it to the bottom of the corner.

toddler's reach, right along with the heavy stuff. Avoid using pedestal tables to hold weighty items.

Use Furniture Padding

Not even a safety advocate like me would tell you to store or get rid of all your furniture, but it is an inescapable fact that every small child bumps into household furniture. Keep the furniture, but cover the corners! You can cushion the bumps and falls by attaching corner and edge guards to all sharp edges on chairs, bookshelves, cabinets, fireplace hearths, and all table and countertops—including that fixture of American living rooms, the coffee table. My husband and I, when our children were toddlers, did something you might consider: we put the coffee table in storage for the first 4 years of our child's life. That can seem like a long time, especially if you have more than one child, but we took that step after our son used the coffee table as a launching pad. He found out he couldn't fly, and we decided we could do without the table.

Windows

Prevent Your Child's Access to Windows

I covered this point in Chapter 1, "Creating a Safe Nursery." To reiterate: Do not keep cribs, chairs, benches, tables, toy boxes, or even a bookcase near the window. Such items are an open invitation for the child to climb up to the window.

Install Window Safety Devices—Don't Depend on Screens

Yes, you've arranged the furniture with safety in mind, but a toddler can get places you never dreamed he could. On average, according to the U.S. Consumer Product Safety Commission, eight children ages 5 and under die each year as a result of falling out of windows, and 3,300 children are injured due to such falls. Avoid a false sense of security; a child can fall from a window that is opened more than 4 inches. Keep your windows closed and locked when children are present.

If possible when you open a window, open it from the top, not the bottom. Do not keep cribs, chairs, benches, tables, toy boxes, or even a bookcase near the window. Such items are an open invitation for the child to climb up to the window. And don't depend on screens. These are no more than flimsy barriers to keep bugs out.

A child can die or be severely injured due to falling from even a first-floor window, so for the best protection against falls, secure every window in your home—especially windows on the second story and above. (If you can't install window safety devices on every window now, prioritize which windows to begin installing them on. Second story and higher windows should be taken care of first.)

Window guards are adjustable metal or aluminum grates with bars no more than 4 inches apart. The guards work with all types of windows and are installed by screwing the guard into the window frame. For windows on the sixth floor and below, you must install window guards that adults and older children can easily open in case of fire. For the seventh floor and above, permanent window guards should be used. Before you make a purchase or install guards, check local building and fire codes.

Window stops are another option, and they cost as little as $2. The device attaches to the inside of the window frame or the upper window to prevent the window from opening more than 4 inches. Some new windows have window stops built into the frame.

Easy-to-install window guards and window stops can be found online and at most hardware and home improvement stores. Make sure the window guards and window stops meet ASTM standards for safety. Follow the manufacturer's instructions to make sure you install the window guards and stops correctly.

Another type of window is the sliding glass door. Herein lies another kind of danger. While your child isn't likely to fall out of it, she can certainly collide with it. To prevent her from crashing into a glass door, thinking it is open, apply large, colorful safety stickers at the child's eye-level. To keep your child safely inside, use a door lock made for sliding glass doors and secure the doors with a bar in the door track. Don't let your children play around sliding glass doors.

Balconies, Decks, and Porches

Keep small children away from balconies, decks, and porches by keeping all access doors locked. Install child-resistant locks on the backyard door. Make sure any children playing in these areas are closely supervised.

DO IT YOURSELF!

Install proper railings.
- Railings should have a minimum height of 42 inches.
- Spaces between the railing and slats should be no wider than 3 ½ inches.
- Install a railing guard made of Plexiglas, plastic, or mesh if spaces are too wide apart. (For outdoor use, make sure materials are designed to withstand the elements, including UV.) Never use safety netting or any railing guard on railings that are spaced too far apart to provide adequate support for the product. If such is the case, remodeling is necessary.

Take Steps to Safeguard Children Near Railings

Even if you are carefully supervising your child, safety measures must always be in place. Do not leave plants, planters, chairs, benches, or any other object that a child could climb up on anywhere near the railing. Be aware that ambitious children may try to move a chair over to the railing to "get a better look." Ensure they cannot do this by using deterrent means appropriate to the object.

Make sure proper railings are in place (see sidebar) and maintain them regularly. Do not allow them to become loose. Never leave your child unattended and do not rely solely on any safety item to keep your child safe.

Garage Door

Because the garage door is the largest moving object in your home, it needs special consideration. A child can suffer permanent brain damage—or die—as a result of an incident involving an automatic door opener.

Not an Option: Install Safety Devices on Your Automatic Door

As of 1991, automatic garage-door openers are required to have an auto-reverse mechanism to reverse the door's direction if it comes in contact with an object. If you have an older opener without an automatic reversal system, it should be replaced immediately. When purchasing a new garage-door opener, make sure it carries the mark of a recognized testing lab such as UL (Underwriters Laboratories) or ETL (Electrical Testing Laboratories).

For further protection, federal law has required that automatic garage-door openers manufactured on or after January 1, 1993, be equipped with an additional entrapment protection feature, such as a photoelectric sensor. This electric eye projects an invisible light beam across the inside of the garage door opening. If anything interrupts the beam while the door is going down, it will automatically reverse the door before making contact. If you don't wish to tackle this project yourself, a company that installs garage-door openers can install these safety devices.

Refer to the manufacturer's instructions for ongoing maintenance of the garage door and operator as well as regular testing of the safety reversing features. Inspect your garage door monthly to see if it is operating properly. If it is not, disconnect the automatic opener from the door (as specified in the owner's manual) and manually open and close the door until it is repaired.

Additional precautions include placing all activation buttons at least 6 feet above the floor, out of the hands of your child. Also, keep the remote control for the door locked in the glove compartment of your car. Do not let it seem to be a toy; do not let a child operate or play with the opener. For home security purposes, always lock the entry to the inside of your home from the garage, especially if your opener is programmed to your vehicle. In addition, always keep your car doors locked.

Don't Take Anything for Granted

Safety devices can fail. Make sure you have a full view of the garage door when you are using the opener. Always check for obstructions—especially live ones such as children and pets. Keep them a safe distance away from the door while it is moving and continue to watch the door until it has completely opened or completely closed. Don't pull out of the driveway until the door has completely shut.

No one should be allowed to run underneath a moving door. That goes for you, too, Mom and Dad! Be role models. Warn your child of the potential dangers of crossing under a moving garage door. Store children's play items away from the garage door, thus removing the temptation to run under a moving door to retrieve something.

Juvenile Equipment

Being careful when you make a purchase is the first step in preventing injuries with baby equipment. Look for the JPMA (Juvenile Products Manufacturer Association) certification label. And when using baby equipment, always follow the manufacturer's instructions on assembly, care, and use. However, there is one piece of equipment we see all the time that is simply not a good choice.

Don't Buy a Wheeled Baby Walker

The American Academy of Pediatrics has long called for the ban of wheeled baby walkers. In fact, baby walkers are banned in Canada. These products are dangerous, and injury risk is high. The most severe injuries are caused when a child falls down stairs with the walker. Even when there are no stairs or when the safety gates are always locked, your child can still tip it over, fall out of it, or reach places where he can pull hot foods or heavy objects down on himself.

Ironically, most walker injuries happen while adults are supervising. You simply cannot respond quickly enough. A child in a walker can move more than 3 feet in 1 second! And despite the name, a baby walker does not help a child to walk earlier. Indeed, some research suggests that use of the walker may delay motor skill development.

Using a stationary activity center is still fun for your baby, and it is a much safer choice. But remember, children like to rock, jump and bounce when they are in one of these centers. For that reason, you should keep it away from hazardous locations, such as stairs, doors, coffee table and TV, and stay with your baby at all times. It's best to use the activity center only for brief periods. Your baby needs the exercise of crawling to develop coordination and strength in her arms and legs.

Stay Vigilant When Using a Changing Table

Buy a changing table or dresser that is sturdy and stable. The American Academy of Pediatrics recommends a 2-inch guardrail around all four sides, with the top of the table being concave, so that the middle is slightly lower than the sides.

Choose a thick, contoured changing pad, with a non-skid bottom. Whether you use a changing table or the top of a dresser, safety restraints are a must. Always use those safety restraints.

Even with safety devices, you need to keep one hand on your baby at all times; never move away, not even for a second. Put diapers and toiletries within your reach before you place that squirming little bundle of joy on the table. At the same time, you have to make sure the items are not within your baby's reach. Most of those objects present a danger if they go into the baby's mouth, and you know where she likes to put things. If she gets her hands on them and doesn't put them in her mouth, she is likely to pitch them, just to make you go fetch. That can be a fun game when she's not in danger of falling off a table, but when you're trying to change her, not so much.

Use a High Chair with a Wide Base, Locks, and Safety Restraints

Select a high chair with a wide, stable base, and test models fitting that description before you purchase. Set your child in each chair you like, making sure the straps fit snugly against her. If she can wiggle out of the strap, it is not tight enough. (I don't think you'll have to tell her to wiggle.) The chair you purchase should have a crotch post, a waist strap, and a crotch strap that are independent of the tray. Many new high chairs are now equipped with a 5-point harness system (waist and crotch restraint with shoulder straps). I highly recommend getting the 5-point harness, because the most common type of injury associated with a high chair is a fall; the shoulder straps on a 5-point harness will keep your baby safely seated. Before you buy, test the safety restraints, choosing ones that are sturdy as well as easy for an adult to fasten and unfasten but secure enough that baby can't open it. Why should it be easy for an adult to manipulate? Because if you have trouble, you'll be tempted not to use the safety devices upon occasion. If it's a folding high chair, make sure it won't pinch fingers when closing.

If the high chair has wheels, the wheels should easily lock in place. Make sure the wheels are locked every single time the high chair holds your child—no exceptions. If you have chosen a folding high chair, make sure it is locked each time you set it up. When you use any high chair, make sure the tray is locked securely in place, but don't rely on it to keep the child from falling out. Always use the safety harness; strap in your baby every single time you use the high chair.

You know the drill by now: Place the chair far away from any table, counter, or wall so your little darling can't use them to push off. Don't allow him to stand on the chair. Stay close.

Millions of unsafe high chairs have been recalled during recent years, so check *recalls.gov* to be sure your high chair is safe. And look for the JPMA certification seal on the packaging.

The American Academy of Pediatrics (AAP) offers an additional caution: A high chair that hooks onto a table is not a good substitute for a freestanding one. If you plan to use this type of chair when you eat out or travel, look for one that locks onto the table. Be sure the table is heavy enough to support your child's weight without tipping. Also, check to see whether your child's feet can touch a table support. If your child pushes against the table, it may dislodge the seat.

Use a Stroller That Will Not Tip and Has Convenient Brakes

A stroller should have a base wide enough to prevent it from tipping, even when your baby leans over to one side. Check the stroller's stability by pressing down lightly on the handles; the stroller should resist tipping backward. It should have a strong, durable, 5-point harness that is easy for you to open and close but difficult for small hands to unbuckle. If there is a shopping basket for carrying items attached to the stroller, the basket should be low on the back of the stroller or be located directly over the rear wheels. Use a stroller that was made for your child's age, height, and weight. If you plan to use a stroller for an infant, make sure the stroller fully reclines, because newborns can't sit up or hold up their heads.

Anything with wheels should have brakes. Stroller brakes should actually lock the wheels and be convenient to operate. Having brakes on two sides provides an extra measure of safety.

In the last decade, millions of strollers have been recalled. As of September 10, 2015, the CPSC has mandated stricter safety standards for newly manufactured strollers, requiring the strollers to be built, tested and labeled to limit hazards. Make sure your stroller meets current national safety standards and is JPMA certified.

Follow Guidelines for Safe Stroller Use

Perhaps the premier safety rule for use of the stroller is never to leave a child unattended, even when he is sleeping, because he can move into a position that can cause him to suffocate. In addition, other children should not be allowed to push it or get into it when the baby is in it. It's probably a good idea just to never let children play with the stroller, even without the baby's presence. The following tips help ensure safe stroller use:

- Before you put the baby in a stroller, use its locking device to prevent unintentional folding.
- Apply the brakes to limit rotation of the wheels when the stroller is stationary, this means when you are putting the baby in or taking her out, or parking it for some reason.
- Secure the safety harness, always! It should fit snugly to keep your child in place.
- Close the leg openings. When used in a reclined position, if the openings are not closed at the crotch, a baby can slip through feet first and become entrapped by his head between the seat and the hand-rest bar. Strangulation could result.
- Don't hang your handbag, diaper bag, or other items over the handles. This can cause even a stable stroller to tip.
- When you fold or unfold the stroller, or when the seat back is being reclined, keep your child away. Small fingers can get caught in stroller hinges.

Check Your Playpen/Play Yard for Dangerous Design Flaws

When selecting a play yard, it's best to buy new. In any case, be sure to use one that was manufactured on or after February 28, 2013 to meet current safety standards. Look for JPMA certification.

In the 1990s, millions of North American play yards—many of them popular brand-name models—were designed with dangerous flaws. In some cases, children died when the top rails collapsed and entrapped their necks. These play yards had a hinge in the center of each top rail that had to be rotated to set up the playpen; if the hinge was not rotated completely, the top rail could collapse and form a V. Play yards made since 1997 have top rails that automatically snap into place and do not need to be rotated when you set up the play yard. Another hazard is protruding rivets. Some toddlers strangled when loose clothing or pacifier strings tied around their neck got caught on the rivets. (Remember, nothing should be tied around a child's neck.)

Select a play yard with a sturdy frame and side rails, and strong corner brackets. It should have a thin, firm mattress that fits tightly and is securely attached to the floor of the play yard. Read the warning label on the play yard; it states to ONLY USE the mattress pad that comes with the play yard. Don't add an extra mattress. Babies can get trapped between the mattress and sides and suffocate. (Although "play yard" mattresses may be sold in some stores, they are never safe to use in mesh sided products.) If you need a replacement mattress for your play yard, contact the manufacturer directly.

Use Your Play Yard Correctly

Even a play yard with a safe design if used inappropriately can harm your child. (Please refer to the safety guidelines outlined in Chapter 1, "Creating a Safe Nursery.") More precautions are noted below:

- Never leave your baby in a mesh play yard with the drop-side down. Babies can suffocate if they roll into the gap between the mattress and the loose mesh side.
- Be especially careful about play yard attachments. Changing tables and bassinet attachments must be carefully installed. (Review warning labels and instruction materials carefully when assembling.)
- Stop using the bassinet when your baby reaches the manufacturer's recommended weight limit (around 15 pounds) or can sit up, pull up, or roll over.
- Never place a baby in the play yard while the change table or bassinet insert is in place.
- When using a sheet, make sure it is tight-fitting and made specifically for the mattress or bassinet insert on your model.
- Only use the mattress pad provided by the manufacturer as directed on the warning label. Never add any additional mattress to the play yard as this is a known suffocation hazard.
- Give it up when the time comes. Do not place a child in a play yard once she has reached 35" tall—about the age of 2—or has become persistent in her efforts to climb out. Be sure to check manufacturer's instructions as to maximum height and weight recommendations.

Remember, for safe sleep in a play yard—just as in a crib and bassinet—bare is best!

Recall Information

Even when you have used the greatest care and looked for appropriate labels, there can still be a product recall. That's one of the reasons you'll want to fill out the registration form. If there is one available for that product, send it to the manufacturer. Only if you are registered can the company notify you of a recall. You can also usually find the online registration form on the manufacturer's website if you don't have a card. Recalls can occur at any stage of a product's life cycle, so you must stay up-to-date regarding everything you use. It is now easier than ever to be informed about recalls. All recalling federal agencies can be found at *www.recalls.gov*. At this link, you can see the latest recalls in consumer products, motor vehicles, boats, food, medicine, cosmetics, and environmental products. Just click on the desired topic.

This is one-stop shopping at its best. For example, if you have purchased a play yard, you can sign up at the site for CPSC recall notices. Of course, you may go to the individual agency websites, too. Those agencies and their websites, along with other ways to contact the agencies, can be found in Appendix D, "Recall Information."

Recall information is also available at *www.KidsInDanger.org*. Download the Children's Product Safety Checklist from the publications page and check all the children's products in your home against the list. On that site you can also sign up for monthly e-mail alerts about recalls and product safety news.

When Bedtime Means a Real Bed

Regardless of construction, a bed is not a safe sleeping or napping area for an infant or any child under 2 years of age. (Please refer to Chapter 1, "Creating a Safe Nursery," for safe sleep recommendations for babies.) Wait until the child is at least 2 years of age before introducing a pillow. Consult your child's pediatrician prior to introducing a bed or pillow to ensure there are no reasons to postpone the introduction. When the pediatrician has given the okay, choose a firm, small pillow.

The safest place for a baby to sleep is in a crib. A toddler should be in his own bed. Infants and toddlers should always sleep or nap alone without siblings or other people. Experts do not recommend co-sleeping or bed-sharing for babies and toddlers.

When Your Toddler Is Ready to Use a Bed, Know the Rules

Because many cribs convert into a toddler bed (and also because children can be moved directly from the crib to a twin bed) it is unnecessary to buy a stand-alone toddler bed. However, if you do purchase a toddler bed, make sure it meets the CPSC's stronger safety standards and is JPMA certified.

Use the same positioning care with the beds as you do with cribs, bassinets and play yards; do not position a "big kid bed" near windows, draperies, window covering cords, electrical cords, baby monitor cords and other cords, nor near hanging wall decorations, heating sources, or climbable furniture.

When your child begins using a twin bed, it's a good idea to put the mattress on the floor. Keep the floor area around the bed clear, and be sure it is in a safe space. No matter the size of the bed, strictly enforce a policy of no playing or jumping on beds.

Portable bed rails are intended for use only on full-size twin beds (with a mattress and box spring) to help prevent children from falling out of bed. *Never* use such bed rails on a toddler bed or bunk bed, because the mattress is too small to support either of them. If you choose to use portable bed rails, your child must be at least 2 years old and able to climb in and out of bed on her own. Carefully follow the manufacturer's instructions on assembly, care, and use. It's important to use two bed rails, one for each side of the bed, even if one side is against the wall. Children can become entrapped and die when they get caught between the bed and wall. Make sure to use portable bed rails that meet the stronger CPSC safety standards issued on February 22, 2012.

Say No to Bunks

Every year nearly 36,000 children suffer injuries related to bunk beds, and children younger than 6 suffer the majority of injuries. A particular hazard for young children is poor depth perception. In addition, they are top-heavy, so when they fall, they are more likely to fall on their head. Don't allow children under the age of 6 to be on the top bed or to play unattended in a room with a bunk bed. Avoid using bunk beds before both children who will be using the bunks are at least 6 years old. Younger children will always try to imitate older siblings, and that will include climbing to the top bunk. When your younger child is ready to use one, make sure the bunk bed meets current safety standards and has not been recalled. Even at age 6, your little daredevil may think pinning a towel around his neck will enable him to fly. Chances are he'll jump head-first. A safety lesson when the bunk beds first arrive and frequent reinforcement are good ideas.

Review and Safety Checklist

- ☑ Use power-failure night-lights at the top and bottom of stairs and throughout your home, particularly in halls, bedrooms, and bathrooms.
- ☑ Install safety gates at the top and bottom of stairs. Do not use a pressure-bar gate at the top of the stairs and keep all gates locked.
- ☑ Arrange furniture in a way that reduces the risk of tipping. Store heavy or breakable items away from little hands.
- ☑ Anchor all large and top heavy furniture and objects securely to the wall, and attach cushioned corner-and-edge protectors on furniture.
- ☑ Install window safety devices on every window in your home, especially windows on the second story and above. Use quick-release mechanisms on any windows that are part of your fire-escape plans. Check local building and fire codes.
- ☑ Install safety devices on your automatic garage door and always watch it to make sure it completely shuts.
- ☑ Don't put your baby in a wheeled baby walker.
- ☑ Make sure all baby equipment meets current safety standards.
- ☑ Use all safety features, such as safety restraints, with all baby equipment, such as the changing table, the high chair, and the stroller. No matter how many restraints and safety features you engage, never leave your child unattended.
- ☑ Stay up to date with recall information.

Safety in the Backyard

If your child can't be safe in her own backyard, where can she be safe? You'll be as excited as she is when she begins to explore the world outside the four walls of your home. She'll learn what fun she can have, just by smelling flowers, hearing birds, seeing butterflies, touching grass, feeling the breeze as it moves her hair in tempo with the branches of trees overhead. She'll also learn about outdoor activities, and it's up to you to make sure those activities do not hurt her.

First make sure your yard itself is safe by fencing it in. If only the backyard is fenced, never allow your child to play in the front yard. Even if you are right there—and you should always be right there, closely supervising your child!—you may not be able to stop a toddler from darting out into the street.

It follows, of course, that children should never play in the driveway. Even when a car is moving slowly, a child that is hit can be seriously hurt or killed. Toddlers can move quickly, have no sense of danger, and may be out of a driver's line of vision simply because of their short stature.

If there are any poisonous plants in your yard, pull them out. (See Chapter 10, "Common Poisons in the Home," and Appendix B, "Common Poisonous Plants.") No matter how beautiful they are, if they can harm your child, you do not want them. You must also take care concerning the pesticides used in your yard. (See Chapter 11, "Environmental Hazards," under the topic "Pesticides," where you'll find safer methods to eliminate pests.)

Yard work is important for safety, no matter what the season. Repair cracks or chips in cement sidewalks and stairs, and keep those stairs and walkways clear of snow, wet leaves, and other debris.

Before we step into the backyard, we'll consider safety in some spaces that are not outside, but which are not usually considered part of your living space: the garage, the workshop, and the basement. This entire chapter is a do-it-yourself project, so get ready for some down-to-earth (and down-to-water) advice.

Garage, Workshop, and Basement

The garage, workshop, and basement are difficult to make safe even for older children, so keep these rooms strictly off-limits to your young child. High dead bolts or flip locks should be in use to prevent the child's entry into these rooms. Even with those locks in place, you must take safety precautions, just in case your child wanders in (perhaps following you).

Start by first inspecting the room and determining what you really want or need to save. Unnecessary items that are not useful should be discarded. It's a good idea to buy only what you will need for each particular project at hand. The savings for quantity is usually not worth buying a special locked cabinet in which to store the extra material safely. For those items you must keep, get a locking storage cabinet.

Use and Store All Tools Safely

Designate specific places for tools and hang them out of reach of children. Having a place for each tool has the added benefit of prompting all the adults with access to the room to return each tool to its proper place after its use. That makes it a snap to find it the next time you want to use it. Wherever you store your power tools, disconnect them when they are not in use.

Take Extra Precautions When Using and Storing Flammable Liquids

All flammable liquids such as gasoline, paint thinners, and kerosene should be kept in properly labeled, tightly closed, safety-approved containers. These products should be stored out of the reach of children, outside the house in a locked shed or detached garage. Keep them in a well-ventilated place away from any source of ignition, and always take the containers outside when fueling power mowers and other equipment. They produce invisible explosive vapors that can be ignited by a small spark at considerable distances from a flammable substance.

Store All Buckets Upside Down

Remember that a small child can drown in as little as 1 inch of water.

Store and Lock Poisonous Products Out of the Reach of Children

All poisons should have child-resistant caps. Keep all products in their original containers and never mix products. Common items you need to lock away, out of the sight and reach of children, are:

- pest-control products
- weed killers and fertilizers
- car-care products such as antifreeze, motor oil, and wind-shield-washer solution
- turpentine, paints, and paint thinner
- pool supplies
- kerosene
- art and hobby supplies
- glues and adhesives
- charcoal lighters

Install Safety Devices

Your automatic garage door should have an auto-reverse device equipped with an additional entrapment protection feature, such as a photoelectric sensor. Install a smoke alarm and carbon monoxide alarm in the basement. (Alarms should be installed on every level of the home.) A carbon monoxide alarm should be installed at least 15 feet from a fuel burning appliance. Carefully follow the manufacturer's installation instructions. As in the rest of the house, you should make sure alarms are working properly and are properly maintained.

Alarms are further considered in other chapters. Please see Chapter 8 regarding smoke alarms and Chapter 11 for a discussion about carbon monoxide. For more information regarding automatic garage openers, please see Chapter 5.

Take Precautions to Prevent Entrapment

Entrapment hazards include:

- clothes dryers
- old style latch-type refrigerators

- latch-type freezers
- combination washer-dryer units
- camper ice boxes
- picnic coolers
- storage chests

Suffocation deaths occur in such places when children crawl inside and cannot escape. The tight-fitting gasket on most appliances cuts off air to the child, and the insulated construction of the appliances prevents anyone from hearing her cry for help.

Take measures to childproof old refrigerators and other appliances that are in storage or are to be discarded. The surest method is to take off the door and leave in the shelves. Keep children away from any currently used item that may present an entrapment hazard by locking the door to the area where it is kept. To keep children from entrapment in your car, make certain it stays locked and the windows are always up.

Keep Your Child Away from Outdoor Power Equipment

Okay, we're almost ready to go outside, but if anyone is using power equipment out there, keep your child indoors and supervised closely at all times. Turn off any power equipment when a child enters a work area. After any outdoor task is complete, store garden tools and other equipment locked out of your child's reach. This goes for mowers and garden tractors, as well as carts or trailers that are pulled behind them. Don't let any child play near a mower, even when it is stationary. Naturally, this proscription is even more important when the mower or tractor is engaged. Such equipment is not a toy; don't let the kids ride on it.

The Outdoors

It is possible that until your child has his first outdoor outing, he has never been bitten or stung by a bug. Another new experience is his exposure to the sun, making him at risk for sunburn. You are certainly in no hurry for him to have any of these experiences. If the weather permits, the best way to protect your child from the sun, bug bites, and ticks is to cover his skin with a hat; a lightweight, long-sleeved shirt; and long pants. Tuck clothing into pants and pant cuffs into socks.

Know What to Do About Ticks

Most tick bites occur during the spring, summer and early fall months (April-September). However, ticks are active and can bite any time the temperature is higher than 40°F. Ticks live in woods and tall grass, so to discourage them from inhabiting your yard, it is important to keep grass cut short and to remove unwanted vegetation around your home. Don't let children brush up against bushes, trees, leaf litter, or shrubs.

Wear light-colored clothing with a tight weave so you can spot ticks more easily and prevent contact with the skin. (For use and guidelines on insect repellents, see the section later in this chapter.) Scan clothes and any exposed skin frequently for ticks while you are outside. After being outdoors—even in your own yard—when the temperature has exceeded 40°F, immediately put your child's clothing in the dryer on high heat for 10 minutes to kill any ticks that might be on them. If clothes have been washed or are damp, an hour may be necessary.

Shower or bathe your children after coming indoors—preferably within two hours—and perform a head-to-toe tick inspection. It's best to use a magnifying glass, because some ticks are very small, about the size of a poppy seed. The CDC recommends that parents check their children for ticks under the arms, in and around the ears, inside the belly button, behind the knees, between the legs, around the waist, and especially in their hair.

When checking yourself, it's helpful to use a hand-held or full-length mirror to view all parts of your body. And remember to check your pets; you can be bitten in your home if a pet brings a tick inside. Contact your local or state health department for more information about ticks and for guidelines concerning the risks of Lyme disease and other tick-borne infections in your geographical area.

Prevent Stings and Bug Bites

Teach your child to move slowly and carefully around insects and dress him in white, beige, or khaki-colored clothing. Bright colors and flowered or floral prints (and scented soaps, lotions, perfumes, or hair sprays) attract bees and other insects. Food aromas attract insects, so don't feed your children outdoors. Other odors attract insects, too, so keep your child away from garbage cans and out of gardens when flowers are in bloom. Do not permit children to go barefoot outside.

Mosquitoes present a greater danger than most other insects, but not all mosquitoes are the same. Different mosquitoes spread different viruses and bite at different times of the day. Mosquitoes that spread chikungunya, dengue, and Zika bite mostly during the day, but they can also bite at night. Mosquitoes that spread West Nile virus are most active from evening to morning.

The use of EPA-approved mosquito repellent is covered in a later section, but there are other ways to avoid mosquito bites. The Centers for Disease Control (CDC) offer specific recommendations, in addition to those already mentioned, for protecting your family:

1. **Cover Up.** When outdoors, wear loose, light colored clothing, including long-sleeved shirts, pants, shoes and socks and hat.
2. **Take Control.** Control mosquitoes inside and outside. Keep bugs outside by having doors and window screens that are tight-fitting and in good repair. Use your air conditioner if you have one.
3. **Eliminate Breeding Places**. At least once a week, empty and scrub, turn over, cover, or throw out items that hold water, such as flower pots, toys, discarded tires, birdbaths, trash containers, pet water bowls and roof gutters. Even bottle caps can hold enough water for mosquitoes to breed. Fix outdoor pipes and leaky faucets. Check inside your home for breeding places, too.

A note about transmission: according to the CDC, Zika virus is transmitted to people primarily through the bite of an infected mosquito. Symptoms are fever, rash, headache, joint pain, conjunctivitis (red eyes), and muscle pain. Zika can also be passed through sex from a person who has Zika to his or her sex partner. Condoms can reduce the chance of getting Zika from sex. Many people infected with Zika won't have symptoms or will have only mild symptoms. However, a pregnant woman, even one without symptoms, can pass Zika to her developing fetus. Zika infection during pregnancy can cause serious birth defects. There is currently no vaccine or specific medicine for Zika. Consult your health care provider for more information, especially before traveling. CDC recommends that pregnant women not travel to areas with Zika outbreaks.

For more information about avoiding bugs that sting and bite, and to stay up-to-date about mosquito-borne diseases such as Zika and West Nile virus in your area, contact your local or state health department and visit *www.CDC.gov.*

Use Caution When Applying Repellents

In areas where insect vector-borne disease is a risk, it may be necessary to use an effective insect repellent to keep you and your child safe. Use an EPA-approved repellent and always follow the recommendations appearing on the product label. The effectiveness of non-EPA registered

DO IT YOURSELF!

Remove ticks.

The Centers for Disease Control and Prevention say if you find a tick attached to your skin, there's no need to panic. Several tick removal devices are available on the market, but a plain set of fine-tipped tweezers will remove a tick effectively. Here are the CDC recommendations for removing a tick:

1. Use fine-tipped tweezers to grasp the tick as close to the skin's surface as possible.
2. Pull upward with steady, even pressure. Don't twist or jerk the tick; this can cause the mouth parts to break off and remain in the skin. If this happens, remove the mouth parts with tweezers. If you are unable to remove the mouth easily with clean tweezers, leave it alone and let the skin heal.
3. After removing the tick, thoroughly clean the bite area and your hands with rubbing alcohol, an iodine scrub, or soap and water.
4. Dispose of a live tick by submersing it in alcohol, placing it in a sealed bag/container, wrapping it tightly in tape, or flushing it down the toilet. Never crush a tick with your fingers.
5. If you or your child develops a rash or fever within several weeks of removing a tick, see your doctor. Be sure to tell the doctor about the recent tick bite, when the bite occurred, and where you most likely acquired the tick.

insect repellents, including some natural repellents, is not known. Before you buy an insect repellent, be sure to look on the label for EPA approval. (Note: The EPA does not recommend any additional precautions for repellent use by pregnant or nursing women. The standard safety tips and directions for use should be followed. If you have questions or concerns, contact your healthcare provider.)

Avoid products that contain both sunscreens and insect repellents, because sunscreen may need to be reapplied more often and in larger amounts than the repellent.

DEET (chemical name N,N-diethyl-meta-toluamide) is the active ingredient in many repellents. It is used to repel biting insects such as mosquitoes and ticks. Insect repellents should not be used at all on babies younger than 2 months, says the American Academy of Pediatrics. Mosquito netting can be used over infant carriers and strollers. Insect repellents containing DEET should be used sparingly on children and only at the lowest effective concentration appropriate for the amount of time the child will be outdoors.

A higher percentage of DEET in a repellent does not mean that your protection is better; just that it will last longer. Products with less than 10% DEET should provide up to two hours of protection. The American Academy of Pediatrics (AAP) recommends that repellents should contain no more than 30% DEET when used on children. Always use insect repellents according to the label directions. In rare cases, some children have experienced adverse effects after application of DEET. Most of the cases of toxicity in children were related to overdose and misuse. Use just enough repellent to cover exposed skin and clothing and avoid over-application.

It is best to have children wear lightweight, long-sleeved shirts and long pants, when possible. To reduce exposure to DEET, apply repellent to the outer surfaces of clothing—I would put it on the clothes before dressing them—rather than to the skin. (Note: DEET can damage certain plastics and some synthetic fabrics such as rayon and spandex). Never use it under clothing. If you apply repellent to your child's exposed skin, use it sparingly. Do not apply repellent directly from the container to your child's skin. Apply it to your hands, then put it on the child. Avoid using it around your child's eyes and mouth and use it sparingly around his ears. Do not put it on the hands of small children or on cuts, wounds, rashes, sunburns, or any other skin condition.

Do not allow young children to apply repellents themselves. After returning indoors, wash your child's treated skin with soap and water, and wash all treated clothing. If you believe you or a child is having an adverse reaction to a repellent, wash the treated area immediately and call poison control or your pediatrician. Store DEET and other repellents locked out of the sight and reach of children.

Alternatives to DEET

Picaridin (KBR 3023), a chemical repellent, is an effective alternative to DEET. It was introduced into the U.S. market in 2005, after being used widely in Europe and Australia for several years. It is a colorless, nearly odorless liquid that provides long lasting protection. Picaridin should not be used on children under 2 months old.

Oil of lemon eucalyptus (OLE), or para-menthane-diol (PMD), is a plant based repellent that is derived from eucalyptus leaves and twigs. In two recent studies, when oil of lemon eucalyptus was tested against mosquitoes found in the U.S. it provided protection similar to repellents with low concentrations of DEET. However, oil of lemon eucalyptus is not recommended for children under the age of 3 years. Be aware that pure oil of lemon eucalyptus (essential oil not formulated as a repellent) is not recommended; it has not undergone similar, validated testing for safety and efficacy and is not registered with EPA as an insect repellent.

The CDC recommends: if you are also using sunscreen, apply sunscreen first and insect repellent second. Note: DEET-containing insect repellents may decrease the SPF of sunscreens by one-third. Sunscreens may increase absorption of DEET through the skin.

Treating clothing and outdoor gear

Permethrin products are intended to be used on items such as boots, pants, socks, and tents for additional protection. Never use permethrin products directly on your skin. Permethrin-treated products repel and kill ticks, mosquitoes, and other arthropods, and the treatment will last after multiple washings. See product information to learn how long the protection will last. If treating items yourself, follow the product instructions carefully. Wash permethrin-treated clothing separately from other clothes.

For more information about EPA registered insect repellents, see Appendix E, "Helpful Resources," and consult your pediatrician.

Don't Let the Sun's Rays Get to Your Child's Skin

Overexposure to the sun's ultraviolet (UV) rays not only causes a painful sunburn but can lead to other serious health problems, including melanoma, a life-threatening form of skin cancer. In fact, serious sunburns at an early age have been associated with melanoma later in life. Moreover, excessive UV exposure can lead to premature aging of the skin, nonmelanoma skin cancers, and immune system suppression. These effects, however, may not appear until later in life.

A child's skin burns more easily than an adult's, and an infant is particularly vulnerable, so infants 6 months and younger should be kept out of direct sunlight altogether. If you can't avoid the sun, make sure your child wears a wide-brimmed hat and lightweight sun-protective long pants and long-sleeved shirt. Keep her stroller or carrier shaded. The AAP says, however, that when protective clothing and shade are not available, parents can apply sunscreen formulated for babies to small areas, such as the infant's face and the back of the hands. Always consult your pediatrician for more information.

Danger in the sun is not limited to the risk of sunburn. Because infant skin does not sweat effectively, a baby is more susceptible to heatstroke. Exposure to the sun may increase the child's risk.

Whenever possible, limit sun exposure for all children during the peak hours of 10 a.m. to 4 p.m., when rays are the strongest. Use sunscreen that is at least SPF 15 and is broad spectrum (protecting from both UVA and UVB rays). Be sure to choose one made especially for babies, which will make an allergic reaction to the sunscreen less likely and will not burn the eyes. If your child is aged 6 months or older, liberally apply the sunscreen to skin that will be exposed before he is dressed—at least 30 minutes before he goes outside. Choose a water-resistant sunscreen. Reapply it every 2 hours, as well as after your child has been in the water or towels off. Consult instructions on the bottle. Use sunscreens all year round and even on cloudy or cool days. UV rays can penetrate the clouds, and it is possible for skin to burn even if neither you nor your child feels warm. Extra precautions should be taken near sand, snow, concrete, or water, which can reflect up to 85% of the sun's damaging rays.

> **DO IT YOURSELF!**
>
> **Play the shadow game.** If your shadow is shorter than you are, you are more likely to sunburn. Any time you are out in the sun with your child, play the shadow game. Soon she will do it on her own, without your prompting. Teach her the next step, too: when the shadow is short, seek shade!

To help choose a sunscreen for your child, The Environmental Working Group performs an annual sunscreen evaluation based on effectiveness and safety. Go to *www.ewg.org/sunscreen/best-kids-sunscreens*.

Make sure there is shade in your backyard. If you don't have trees that will do the job, you can create your own shade using tents or canopies. Clothing that covers your child's skin helps protect against UV rays, so have her wear a hat and lightweight, long-sleeved, full-length clothing when possible and practical. Cotton fabrics are a good choice, and it's best to use a tightly woven fabric—one that when held up to the light, little shines through. Look for wide-brimmed hats that shade your child's face, scalp, neck, and ears. Consult your pediatrician at once if an infant under the age of 1 is sunburned, or if any of these symptoms are present: a fever, fluid-filled blisters, or pain.

Remember That Sunglasses Are As Important As Sunscreen

Long-term exposure to UV radiation increases the risk of sight-stealing conditions such as cataracts and macular degeneration. Children are more susceptible to UV exposure than adults because the lens in their eyes is clearer. As one ages, the lens yellows and tends to block more

UV to the back of the eye. The feature you should demand when you choose sunglasses is that they have 100 percent UVA and UVB protection. There are a variety of sizes to fit a baby as young as 6 months; don't buy toy sunglasses. Like sunscreen, sunglasses need to be worn on cloudy days as much as on sunny days.

Home Playground Equipment

Keeping your child safe can be tricky if you want to have playground equipment right in your own backyard. It is a sad fact that each year about 200,000 children are treated in U.S. hospital emergency rooms for playground-equipment-related injuries. (An estimated 51,000 involve home playground equipment.) About 15 children die each year as a result of playground-equipment-related incidents; half of the deaths are related to home play settings. Most of these injuries are the result of falls, and most of the deaths reported each year are due to strangulation.

However, there are guidelines to help you make sure your child does not suffer a serious injury and can still have fun. Before allowing your child to touch any play equipment, check for hot surfaces. Hot metal from which you quickly draw your hand away can seriously burn your child's delicate skin. Do not let him play on that equipment.

Get Playground Equipment That Is Right for Your Child's Age and Weight

Don't buy equipment expecting your child to grow into it. If the child is too small for the equipment, he cannot safely use it. Many injuries of young children occur when they play on equipment designed for older children. How do you know if the equipment isn't suitable? If your child cannot reach or use the equipment by himself, it is wrong for him. Start with age-appropriate equipment and add to it in stages, as the child grows. Swing sets should be composed of soft materials, such as canvas or rubber, and no more than two swing seats should be suspended in one section. The American Society for Testing and Materials (ASTM) sets standards for playground equipment. No matter what equipment you buy, be sure it has an ASTM F 1148 label.

Choose the Site Carefully and Install According to the Manufacturer's Instructions

As you plan your yard, keep spacing in mind. Find a place in your yard that is at least 6 feet from walls and at least 7 feet from electrical wires.

(The wires should not go over the playground.) Prepare this area so that it is nearly level but will drain. Follow carefully the manufacturer's instructions for installation and anchor the equipment well. Each single apparatus should be set at least 12 feet from every other structure. Many backyards don't have this much space. If you purchase a home that has playground equipment already installed, be sure the site meets the above requirements.

Several times every month, inspect your playground. Look for splintering, cracks, or signs of wear. Sand wood and put preservative on it annually. Be sure bolts are tight and every piece of equipment is anchored properly. If any equipment is broken, repair it or remove it. Rake the surfacing and remove debris, then check the surfacing depth. Loose-fill playground surfacing should be 12 inches deep. Add more surfacing where necessary.

Provide a Soft Landing

Install a cushioning product over an adequate fall zone. The material should be under and around every swing, every slide every piece of equipment. It should reach at least 6 feet in all directions from each stationary apparatus. For swings, it should extend—at the front and back—as far as twice the height of the suspending bar. Twelve inches of loose fill material such as sand, pea gravel, wood products, or loose rubber products will make a soft-enough cushion, but you can also use rubber or synthetic mats, which require less maintenance. All surfacing, including rubber and synthetic mats must be tested by the ASTM F 1292 standard. (Make sure you see the results in order to know how thick the mat needs to be in relation to the height of the equipment.) Do not use asphalt, concrete, dirt, grass, or soil; they are not safe. Whatever material you use, maintain both the surface and the equipment on a regular basis.

Don't be tempted to get plastic play sets or climbing equipment for indoor use, either, without providing a soft landing. Surfaces such as wood, tile, or cement floors, even if they are carpeted, cannot absorb enough shock from a fall. Plastic play sets and any climbing equipment should be used on shock-absorbing playground surfaces (such as rubber mats) that meet ASTM F1292 standards to prevent head injuries.

Limit the Height of Play Equipment

Limiting the height of play equipment is a primary way to prevent severe injuries from falls. For preschool children, the highest rung or platform on any climbing equipment or the top of a slide should be 4 feet or lower. Provide equipment that has openings less than 3 1/2 inches or more than 9 inches. The spaces between ladder rungs present the most common entrapment hazards, but the openings in guardrails or platforms should also be measured. Children usually go through an opening feet first. If the space is big enough for a child's body but too small for his head, he could strangle.

Dress Your Child in Playground-Safe Clothes

Do not let your child wear anything around her neck that might snag on equipment. This includes oversize clothing, as well as necklaces or scarves. Remove drawstrings from outer attire. In cold weather, use neck-warmers instead of scarves. Closed-toe shoes, such as sneakers, are safe; sandals are not. However, you must make sure laces are tied well enough that they will not come loose and trip the child or get caught in play structures. Do not allow your child to wear a bicycle helmet while on playground equipment. It can get caught on equipment and cause strangulation. A jump rope is also dangerous on the playground. Do not attach a rope to playground equipment and make sure none of the children in your yard use a rope on the playground equipment.

Conversely, be sure there are no points on the play equipment that can catch a child's clothing. A child can strangle to death if he becomes entangled in small spaces. Check especially the top of slides, the S-hooks on swings, and the joints of climbers.

Help Your Child Learn the Rules of Playground Safety by Showing Her How to Use the Equipment

Even in your own backyard, there must be safety rules, and you'd rather your child not learn them the hard way. Make sure your child uses any equipment the way it was intended to be used. Make sure she knows how to do it, and explain the dangers of not following the rules. At first she won't understand, but by following the example you set when you are with her, she'll learn almost automatically.

- When someone else is on the swing, walk far behind it.
- Do not play close to a moving swing.
- Do not play at the bottom of a slide.
- Etiquette is good to practice as well: Wait your turn, and don't push or shove.

Supervise!

Be an active supervisor. Stay close to your child and watch as she plays. This requires your full attention.

Note: Playground equipment is made for children at three different age stages: 6-23 months, 2-5 years, and 5-12 years. Playground equipment for public use (at child care centers, schools, and parks) should meet the standards set by ASTM F 2373 for the youngest stage (6-23 months) and by ASTM F 1487 for the two older stages (2-5 and 5-12 years).

Playground equipment in eating establishments follows the ASTM F 1918 (soft, contained play equipment) standard.

The Family Barbecue

There will come a day when the youngest member of your family is roaming around the yard at a family barbecue. You have already made sure the grill was put together according to the manufacturer's instructions, and you are following your owner's manual regarding the way you use it. Now exercise caution. Your child will be attracted to the smell and sight of food cooking, and because the grill is relatively low to the ground, it is within his reach. Never leave a heated grill unattended and always carefully supervise your child around it. Keep pets, as well as children, away from the grill, especially when it is lit and for hours after, while it is still hot to the touch. With all that, you must also be alert to using the grill with food safety in mind.

Keep Children at Least 3 Feet Away From a Hot Grill

Establish a 3-foot zone, but just in case adults become distracted, the child should be taught never to touch hot coals—make that *any* coals. They may look cool, but coals stay hot long after they have become gray in color. Keep matches, lighter fluid, charcoal, propane, electrical starters, and cooking utensils out of reach. Also, lock the grill when not in use.

Remember the Importance of Bacteria Control in Cooking

Watching out for harmful bacteria is just as important outside as it is in the kitchen. It is a good idea to have two sets of barbecue tongs, so that the one used for putting the raw meat on the grill is not used for taking cooked meat off. Of course, if you have only one set, you can wash the tongs thoroughly while the meat is cooking.

The Swimming Pool

A swimming pool may provide family fun and exercise, but it is one of the most dangerous single areas inside or outside your house. A fact stated in Chapter 4, "Bathroom Safety," is worth repeating here: drowning is the leading cause of injury death for children ages 1 to 4, and the second leading cause of injury death among children ages 1 to 14, according to the CDC.

Install Safety Devices to Restrict Access to the Pool

The more "layers of protection"—barriers and devices—the better, to prevent unsupervised access. Drowning occurs most often when children get access to the pool during a short lapse in adult supervision. A young child can leave the home unnoticed, slipping into the backyard and into the pool.

The best safety device is a four-sided isolation pool fence. Studies show four-sided isolation fencing around home pools could prevent 50 percent to 90 percent of childhood drownings and near-drownings. The fence should be at least 4 feet high, with no footholds, around the entire perimeter of the pool. Safe pool fencing is designed so that children cannot climb over, under or through. Do not use the house as one of the sides, since access to the pool from the house is a major factor in drowning incidents. In addition, the fence should be completely separate from the play area and yard.

(This includes larger portable and inflatable pools that are not emptied after use; it is imperative to install a four-sided isolation pool fence around these pools, too.)

Another important safety feature, a must for your pool, is a system of gates and latches. Only gates that are self-closing and self-latching will do. That way you'll never wonder if you locked the gate—and you'll never forget! The latch function is defeated if you prop open the gate to the pool area. Don't let anyone do that, including service people. If a pool or lawn care company comes to your home, emphasize to the manager, as well as to the technician, the importance of always securing the pool gate.

All gates should open away from the pool, and their latches should be out of reach of children. Move furniture away from the fence so your child can't climb up to reach the latch or climb over the fence. Inspect the gates and latches often and be sure they are in good working order. All doors in the home—not just the gates on the pool fence—should have child-resistant locks and be self-closing, if possible. Install window guards or window stops (see Chapter 5, "Preventing Falls in the Home").

Installing audible alarms on the doors and windows, which will let you know when someone leaves the house, will notify you when your child goes outside and might be heading for the pool. Adding a pool alarm is also recommended.

In conjunction with a pool fence, an automatic pool cover (a motorized cover operated by a switch) may be used to add protection. The cover should meet the requirements of the American Society for Testing and Materials (ASTM). ASTM requires that a cover be able to withstand the weight of two adults and a child so that a rescue is possible should an individual fall onto the cover. (Note: Manual covers are a less costly option. They should also meet ASTM standards. However, the ASTM and the CPSC do not recommend that manually operated pool covers act as a standalone layer of protection. Use only in conjunction with a pool fence.) Be aware that solar/floating pool covers are *not* safety devices. As with all other pool equipment, you will want to follow the manufacturer's directions for safe use, installation, and maintenance. When the cover is in place, keep it locked, and never leave a pool cover partially in place; a child can be trapped underneath. Here's that reminder again: A child can drown in an inch of water! Keep that in mind and drain any standing water from the surface of the cover.

Make Sure the Pool Is Safe

Read and carefully follow all operating and maintenance instructions furnished by the pool manufacturer, as well as those for pool equipment and chemicals. Remember to store pool supplies and chemicals locked out of the sight and reach of children. Even when you're sure you're doing everything right, inspect the pool and equipment regularly. If you find anything amiss, have a professional make any necessary repairs.

In the pool, as in the bathroom or anywhere else in the home, water and electricity do not mix! Keep electrical appliances (including telephone wire) away from the pool and make sure any electrical outlets near the pool are covered. If an appliance must be near the pool, make sure it has a ground fault circuit interrupter. If at all possible, use battery-operated appliances. On the subject of electricity: Don't allow swimming during a thunderstorm. Swimming during inclement weather should be forbidden always, but this is so especially when there is lightning.

Routinely inspect drain and suction outlet covers to be sure they are in place and are not cracked or missing. A missing, askew, or broken cover can cause serious injury or death to children because of the drain's strong suction action. If drains are used, dual drains are recommended. This minimizes the suction of any one drain, reducing risk of death or injury. Replace drain covers with anti-entrapment covers. Without such covers, a person can be held underwater when her hair, an arm, a leg, or part of her torso becomes entrapped in the drain. Do not allow your child in any type of pool or hot tub/spa unless it is equipped with a securely attached anti-entrapment drain cover, and teach your child to stay away from drains. Show everyone where the cutoff switch for the pump is located, just in case. Any swimmer with long hair should tie it up or wear a bathing cap to prevent becoming entangled in a drain cover. An even better idea: cut your child's hair for the summer; it's safer in the pool and cooler at poolside. Install a safety vacuum release system to automatically release the vacuum should an entrapment occur. Note: The Virginia Graeme Baker Pool and Spa Safety Act (VGBA) is a federal law that requires public pools and spas to have safer and compliant drain covers to avoid entrapment hazards.

The deck, too, can present hazards. In addition to keeping electrical appliances away from the pool area, any breakable objects such as glass should not be used. The deck should be clear of any objects that children may trip over.

Learn These Lessons for Life

Teach children how to swim. Every child is different, so enroll children for swimming lessons when they are ready. Consider age, development and how often they are around water. (If you're thinking of enrolling your child in a swim class, the American Academy of Pediatrics recommends first talking it over with your child's pediatrician to find out if your child is developmentally ready for it.)

No matter what class you enroll yourself and your child in, make sure the instructor is certified. There are many free or reduced-cost options available; among them are those offered by your local YMCA, USA Swimming Chapter, the Parks and Recreation Department, and the local Red Cross Chapter. Also make sure classes are conducted in pools that comply with current standards for design, maintenance, operation, and infection control.

The America Academy of Pediatrics states there is no scientific evidence that swim programs can teach self-rescue skills to infants less than 1 year of age. Swim programs for babies should focus solely on providing a fun activity for babies with their parents. Swim programs must not be expected to "drown-proof" a child of any age; adults should closely supervise all children in or near water, even those who are strong swimmers. And use additional layers of protection that include pool fencing, supplemental pool alarms and rigid covers, and the constant use of life jackets.

Always—Carefully and Constantly—Supervise Your Child Around Water

As mentioned above, there is no such thing as "drown-proof." Constant eye contact and active supervision is required when children are in and around water. Never leave them alone, not for one second. Any time children are in or around water, a responsible adult must be there, watching carefully. Don't multitask while supervising: no reading, napping, texting, talking on the telephone, or taking care of another child. The adult who supervises should know how to swim and know how to administer CPR. The American Academy of Pediatrics recommends that whenever infants or toddlers are in or around water, an adult should be within arm's length, providing "touch supervision."

Do not use air-filled swimming aids or foam toys in place of life jackets or life preservers. Such aids can give parents and children a false sense of security, which may increase the risk of drowning. These are toys and are not designed to be personal flotation devices. Remember, no device is a substitute for adult supervision.

Children should always wear a properly sized U.S. Coast Guard approved personal safety device around oceans, rivers, and lakes, and always when participating in water sports. During social gatherings, designate an adult as a "Water Watcher," a supervisor whose sole responsibility is to constantly observe children in and around water. (It's helpful if adults take turns paying undivided attention, such as for 15-minute periods.) When parents become preoccupied, children are at risk. (Unfortunately, many drownings occur at pool parties with many adults present—everyone thinks someone else is watching, when, in reality, no one is watching.) When swimming at public swim areas, allow your child to swim only if there is a lifeguard, but do not rely on that person to personally supervise your child. The lifeguard has too many children to watch to be able to give one child individual attention.

Safety can often be a matter of good manners. Teach your children never to run, push, or jump on others around water.

Take Precautions after the Swim

Teach your children to take all their toys out of the pool at the end of pool time. Make sure all toys have been removed so there will be no enticement—in addition to the water itself—for the child to want to return to the pool area. Before leaving the area, make sure the gate and pool cover are locked. Keep other playthings and tricycles away from the pool area all the time; a playing child could fall in. To signal that pool time is over, take off your child's swimsuit immediately after the swim. If the pool is portable or inflatable, empty it each and every time following use and place a tamper-proof cover over it, or turn it upside down (to avoid the accumulation of rain water). Store the pool out of children's reach. For an aboveground pool or an inflatable pool with a ladder, remove the steps before leaving the area.

Be Prepared for an Emergency

Learn infant/child CPR and first aid and have your babysitters and anyone else who cares for your child learn it, too. In addition, instruct caregivers about potential hazards to your child in and around swimming pools, impressing upon them the need for constant supervision. Keep these rescue equipment items near the pool: a U.S. Coast Guard approved life preserver and ring buoy, with a line securely attached, and a long-handled hook to assist or retrieve a victim from the water. Also, keep first aid kits on hand and post CPR instructions near the pool.

Keep a phone at poolside, so you won't be wasting precious time in an emergency. Have emergency contact numbers programmed into the phone. (See the "Form for Emergency Numbers" in Appendix F.)

Make an emergency plan. The first step is having a clear view of the pool from your home, even if it requires the removal of trees, bushes, or other obstacles. If you ever turn around and find that your child is missing, every second counts. Before you look anywhere else, check your pool or spa. If a child is missing from the pool area, check the pool first. Go to the edge of the pool and carefully scan the entire body of water, bottom and surface, as well as the surrounding pool area.

DO IT YOURSELF!

Practice good hygiene.
- Don't allow your child to swim when she has diarrhea. This is especially important for kids in diapers. They can spread the germs into the water and make other people sick.
- Don't depend on swim diapers or swim pants. They may hold in some feces, but they are not leak-proof.
- Always wash your child thoroughly (especially his bottom) before swimming. We all have invisible amounts of fecal matter on our bottoms that end up in the pool.
- Teach your child not to drink or swallow water from a pool or any recreational waters.
- Take your child on bathroom breaks or check diapers often to lessen the chance of a fecal accident in the water.
- Make sure you and all family members bathe or shower with soap and water before and after swimming. Thoroughly wash your child's hands, as well as your own, with soap and water after using the bathroom or changing diapers.
- Diaper changing—and checking diapers—should be performed in the bathroom or diaper changing area, never at poolside.
- Stay out of the water if you have an open wound that is not covered with a secure, waterproof bandage.

Become familiar with the pools in your neighborhood. Inspect all of them, as well as those at the homes of relatives or friends whom you frequently visit. Make sure they are properly fenced off and the gates are kept locked.

Take the Same Safety Precautions with Hot Tubs and Spas

Hot tubs and spas can be as dangerous for children as swimming pools and should be regarded with the same degree of caution. Apply the same important safety rules you've read above. In addition, a locked safety cover should be used for your spa. Some non-rigid covers, such as solar covers, can allow a small child to slip into the water while the cover appears to be still in place.

A young child should not use a hot tub or spa, for her lighter body weight and developing organs make her much more sensitive to the stress caused by higher water temperature. The water in a spa is hot enough to damage her delicate skin, as well. Consult with a pediatrician before allowing any child to use the hot tub. In addition, anyone sensitive to high temperatures should consult a physician before using a hot tub or spa. This includes pregnant women, diabetics, heart patients, or anyone taking prescription medicine.

Spa temperatures should never exceed 104º F.

Follow the Rules for Healthy Swimming

Never allow your child to swim in any recreational water that does not meet health standards. Fecal accidents can result in the spread of infectious disease. Germs such as cryptosporidia can survive for days in chlorinated water, and *E. coli* 0157:H7 bacteria are killed only if chlorine is at proper levels. If your child accidentally swallows contaminated pool water, he can become infected. These germs can cause stomachaches and diarrhea; in some cases, they can be deadly.

Review and Safety Checklist

- ☑ Keep your garage, workshop, and basement off-limits for your child, and use high dead bolts or flip locks to help enforce the rule.
- ☑ Store flammable liquids such as gasoline in safety-approved containers outside the home, in a well-ventilated, locked shed or detached garage and away from any source of ignition.
- ☑ Keep poisons, such as antifreeze and windshield-wiper fluid, locked away out of the sight and reach of children.
- ☑ Lock up or remove entrapment hazards, such as coolers and storage chests, and store all buckets upside down.
- ☑ Keep children away from outdoor power equipment.
- ☑ Keep grass cut short, remove unwanted vegetation, and get rid of stagnant water around your home.
- ☑ Perform a head-to-toe tick inspection on your child after every outing when the temperature has exceeded 40ºF.
- ☑ Use caution when applying repellents, carefully following label instructions. Do not use repellents on babies younger than 2 months.

☑ When possible and practical, protect your child from bug bites, ticks, and sunburn by dressing her in brimmed hats; lightweight, long-sleeved shirts; and long pants (avoiding bright or floral patterns). Tuck clothing into pants and pant cuffs into socks.

☑ Infants 6 months or younger should be kept out of direct sunlight. For children over 6 months of age, liberally apply sunscreen with an SPF of at least 15, at least 30 minutes before your child goes out. Use sunscreen and sunglasses (with 100 percent UV protection) year-round, even on cloudy or cool days.

☑ When purchasing and installing playground equipment, make sure it is appropriate for your child's age and weight. Choose the playground site carefully, and provide soft landing material beneath and around all equipment.

☑ Dress your child in clothing that is safe for the playground (nothing loose or dangling), and teach your child the rules of playground safety.

☑ Keep children at least 3 feet away from a hot barbeque grill.

☑ If you have a home swimming pool, install a 4-sided isolation fence at least 4 feet high and equipped with self-closing, self-latching gates. Prevent direct access from a house or yard to the pool or spa.

☑ Install pool equipment according to the manufacturer's instructions and inspect and repair equipment on a regular basis. Take special care with the pool drains; use anti-entrapment covers.

☑ Never leave a child unsupervised in or around water, and never rely on any pool flotation device or swimming lessons to protect a child.

☑ Learn CPR and keep rescue equipment, a phone, and emergency numbers poolside.

☑ After every session in the pool, remove all toys, lock all latches, and drain inflatable and portable pools. Store them upside down.

☑ Take the same safety precautions with hot tubs and spas as you do with swimming pools. In addition, do not allow a young child to use a hot tub or spa.

Safety with Pets

The only little bundle that might come close to warming your heart as much as your baby does is a squirmy puppy or a soft kitten. A child can learn some wonderful life lessons while caring for a pet, but there are potential hazards that accompany pets of any kind. A very young child can harm your pet, and a pet can most certainly harm your child. If you have both a baby and a cat or dog, never leave them in a room alone together. If you do not have a pet already in your home when your first baby is born, postpone getting one—for the sake of the pet, as well as your child. It's best to wait until your child is at least 5 years old before getting a pet. Children under 5 will not always understand or remember instructions. In any case, always make sure you take your time, choosing a pet carefully. Supervise children around pets and teach children how to act around other animals. You can prevent injuries by careful choice, supervision, and education.

Steps to Take If You Already Have a Pet

If you already have a pet in the household, I highly recommend that you consult both your veterinarian and your pediatrician about specific concerns.

Work with a Veterinarian

Regular veterinary visits for your pets are important for the health and safety of everyone in your family. Dogs and cats should be appropriately immunized and kept on flea-, tick-, and worm-control programs.

Keep Your Pet from Causing Injury

- Spay or neuter your dog. Not only will the pet have fewer health problems associated with its reproductive system, but she will also be calmer and less likely to bite.
- Enroll your dog in an obedience training class. (Ask your veterinarian for recommendations.)
- Trim your dog's nails regularly and keep your cat's nails trimmed short and dull.
- Keep your pet's food, water, and toys away from your child. Not only can pet food be a choking hazard, but ingesting some pet foods may be a health hazard for children. The water dish is a drowning hazard. Remember, if it has an inch of water, your child could drown in it. The pet's toys have germs, and even if your baby doesn't put them in her mouth—fat chance!—she'll get the germs on her hands, which will, without a doubt, go in her mouth.
- Avoid using chemical tick and flea collars or flea dips. Choose nontoxic alternatives.

If You Already Have a Dog, Prepare Him for Your Baby's Arrival

Nearly half the dog bites seen in emergency departments have happened with the family pet in the child's own home. That's why it is very important to take steps to prepare your dog for the newborn's arrival.

- Get the dog used to baby sounds before the infant arrives. Prepare a recording of a baby crying (your friends can help with this), and play it for the dog.
- Consider using a toy baby doll to help your dog get accustomed to a real baby. Engage in routine activities, such as feeding, diaper changing, and holding the "baby." Take the dog out for a walk with the doll in a stroller to find out how he will react. You'll have time before the baby comes to teach the dog to behave appropriately.
- Before the baby comes home from the hospital, allow the dog to sniff items the baby has used, such as an undershirt or blanket. That way the dog will become familiar with the baby's smell and be less curious when the newcomer arrives.

DO IT YOURSELF!

Safety Check
- Never leave a baby or young child alone with any pet.
- Keep the baby's room off-limits to your pet. Install a safety gate or screen door.
- Always supervise children around dogs, cats, and other animals.
- Keep a pet's food, water, and toys away from your child.
- Keep all pet supplies locked away and out of children's sight and reach.

If You Already Have a Cat, There Are Some Facts You Should Know

Even before your baby is born, your cat may be a potential source of harm. Your cat or kitten can bring into your home a disease called toxoplasmosis, a flu-like illness caused by a parasite named *Toxoplasma gondii.* Generally known to be transmitted through raw meat—especially pork—toxoplasmosis can also be transmitted through cat feces. If you are healthy and do not have an immune disorder, you can have the disease without knowing it because the symptoms can be mild. If you are pregnant and become infected with toxoplasma for the first time, during or just before your pregnancy, you can pass the infection on to your baby. The disease can cause birth defects such as intellectual disability, liver and spleen damage, and visual impairment or blindness, especially if the fetus becomes infected in the first trimester.

For more information about toxoplasmosis, contact your health care provider. Consult the veterinarian to learn more about your cat's risk for toxoplasmosis. To help prevent your cat from becoming infected with toxoplasma, always keep indoor cats inside. Feed cats dry or canned commercial cat food. Never feed cats raw meat, which can be a source of toxoplasma infection.

Safe Practices Around Animals
Teach Your Child How to Act Around Animals

Even if your home doesn't have a pet, teach your children these safety tips for when they are around animals in others' homes.

DO IT YOURSELF!

Guard against toxoplasmosis.
- If you already have a cat, clean your cat's litter box with care.
- If you are pregnant, let your spouse do it!
- If you are pregnant and must change the litter box yourself, wear gloves and change the box on a daily basis. The parasite found in cat feces needs only 1 day after being passed to become infectious.
- Immediately wash hands thoroughly with soap and water after cleaning the litter box.
- If possible, avoid contact with soil and sand. If you must have such contact, wear gloves when gardening and handling sand from a sandbox. Wash hands well afterwards.
- Follow all food safety guidelines outlined in Chapter 3, "More about the Kitchen."

Always . . .
- treat animals with kindness and respect
- handle pets gently
- wash your hands thoroughly after handling pets

Never . . .
- approach any unfamiliar animal
- disturb an animal that is eating, sleeping, caring for its young, or guarding something
- touch any pet before asking its owner if it is okay to do so
- tease, chase or stare at an animal
- grab an animal by the feet, ears, or tail
- touch or pick up a wild or stray animal
- try to break up animals fighting
- play with a dog unless supervised by an adult

Also show your child what to do if approached by an unfamiliar dog:
- be still like a statue if a dog comes up to you
- if you're knocked down by a dog, roll into a ball and lie still like a rock

Turn this lesson into a game by role-playing.

Practice Sanitation and Good Hygiene

Animals can be a source of illness for people, and people may be a source of illness for animals. Following basic sanitation practices is essential to maintain the safest possible environment for both the pets and the children in your care.

- Everyone—children and adults—should wash their hands after handling pets, pet foods, or pet wastes. Thorough hand washing with soap for at least 20 seconds using clean, running water has been effective in preventing disease transmission.
- Keep pets and their living quarters squeaky clean. Dispose of animal waste immediately. Animal cages should be of an approved type with removable bottoms for easy cleaning.
- Clean up animal feces in the yard immediately. Keep the cat's litter box out of a child's reach and cover children's sand boxes when not in use to prevent cats from using them as litter boxes.

Watch for Ticks

Ticks carrying Lyme disease can be carried into the house by any pet that is allowed outside. Any animal that gets into your yard can carry ticks. Your household pets cannot directly transmit Lyme disease to anyone in your family, but loose, infected ticks on pets can be a hazard for people around them. Ask your veterinarian for advice about which tick control product is best for your pet. For more information about ticks, see Chapter 6, "Safety in the Backyard."

Keep the Fish Tank Off-Limits

Put the fish tank in a place where children cannot climb up on it, fall in it, or pull the tank over on themselves. Secure heavy tanks to the wall with anchoring devices such as safety straps.

Remove Pet Reptiles and Amphibians from Your Home

Reptiles such as iguanas and turtles, and amphibians such as frogs, toads, newts and salamanders, have become popular as household pets, even though these creatures are particularly likely to carry Salmonella bacteria. *Salmonella* is normally in the digestive tract of healthy reptiles and amphibians, but it can cause infections in people who have contact

---

DO IT YOURSELF!

Keep your pet clean.
- Regularly wash pet bedding, rugs, carpets, and furniture coverings.
- Vacuum often—everywhere the pet has gone.
- Bathe your pet and its sleeping areas regularly.
- Clean cat litter trays daily and keep out of the reach of children.
- Dispose of pet waste immediately.

---

with reptiles and amphibians and their environments—including the water from terrariums or aquariums where they live.

Most healthy adults and older children who are infected with Salmonella will recover within a week from its diarrhea, fever, and abdominal cramps without any lasting side effects. However, infants, young children, and anyone with a suppressed immune system is likely to suffer severe or fatal illness from such an infection. These bacteria can be transmitted easily to children through a reptile's or amphibian's feces, which may stick to its body or cage. Without careful hygiene—washing hands thoroughly with soap and water after handling the amphibian or reptile or after cleaning its cage—the fecal material can be ingested or can contaminate any items (such as a pacifier) with which the child's mouth or hands come in contact.

Because of the danger, children under 5 years of age and people with weak immune systems should avoid contact with reptiles and amphibians. In fact, if an infant is going to be brought into the home, reptiles and amphibians should be removed before the newcomer arrives. Practice extra caution when children under 5 visit farms and have direct contact with farm animals, including animals at petting zoos and fairs.

Obviously, neither reptiles nor amphibians should be in child care centers. (Other pets to avoid for children under age 5 are chicks, ducklings or other baby birds. Young birds often carry Salmonella.)

Completely Avoid Having Certain Exotic Animals as Pets

Avoid exotic pets such as monkeys, spiders, and venomous or aggressive snakes, as well as wild animals such as raccoons, bats, and skunks. Your veterinarian or doctor can answer questions about any pet health risks for children and adults in your family.

> ## DO IT YOURSELF!
>
> **Learn to recognize the signs of rabies.**
> You cannot tell if an animal has rabies just by looking at it, but there are signs of rabies that can alert you. *Be suspicious if . . .*
> • a wild animal appears tame
> • a nocturnal animal is seen in the daytime
> • any animal exhibits nervous or aggressive behavior
> • any animal is foaming at the mouth or drooling excessively

Prevent Rabies

Rabies is a serious viral disease that attacks the brain and other nervous system tissue. Although it is almost always fatal if left untreated, the good news is that immediate protective treatment (thorough cleaning of the wound and the vaccine regimen) is effective in preventing the disease from developing. It is true that common carriers are wild animals such as skunks, bats, foxes, and raccoons, but dogs and cats can be infected with rabies, too. Any infected mammal can transmit rabies to humans, either through a bite or by the animal's saliva or nervous tissue entering the human's open wound or mucus membrane (that is, eyes, nose, or mouth). To help protect your family from rabies, be sure to vaccinate your dogs and cats against it. (Ferrets need to be vaccinated, too.) Avoid contact with wild animals and unfamiliar dogs and cats. Do not feed or handle wild animals or strays. Report strays and wild animals that appear sick to your local animal control agency so that they can be captured. Teach your children to enjoy watching wildlife from afar.

Take Immediate Action If a Family Member Is Bitten or Scratched by an Animal

If your child or any family member is bitten or scratched by any animal, act quickly. Wash the wound thoroughly with soap and water for at least 5 minutes and seek medical attention immediately.

If it is a pet that bites or scratches, the animal should be confined and observed for signs of rabies for 10 days. If a wild animal bites or scratches someone, animal control may need to euthanize the animal to test its brain for rabies.

Be aware that a bat does not always leave a bite mark. If you see a bat in a room with your child, seek medical attention. Whenever possible, the bat should be safely captured and sent to a laboratory for rabies testing. Contact your health department or local animal control on the proper procedure for safely capturing a bat found in one's home.

Review and Safety Checklist

- ☑ Wait until your child is 5 years old before getting a pet.
- ☑ Never leave a baby or young child alone with any pet.
- ☑ If you have a pet, regular veterinary visits are important for the health and safety of everyone in your family. Dogs and cats should be appropriately immunized and kept on flea-, tick-, and worm-control programs.
- ☑ Keep the baby's room off-limits to your pet. Install a safety gate or screen door.
- ☑ Always supervise children around dogs, cats, and other animals.
- ☑ If you are pregnant and must change the litter box yourself, wear disposable gloves and change the box on a daily basis. Wash hands thoroughly afterward.
- ☑ Remove pet reptiles and amphibians from a household where children under 5 years old reside.
- ☑ Completely avoid certain exotic animals as pets.
- ☑ Stay away from strays and report them to your local animal control agency.
- ☑ Teach your child to enjoy watching wildlife from afar.
- ☑ Take immediate action if a family member is bitten or scratched by an animal.

Fire Safety

Every year in the United States, more than 2,500 people lose their lives in residential fires. Don't become part of those statistics. Take a 4-step approach to fire safety at home:

- remove potential fire hazards and correct unsafe practices
- install and maintain smoke alarms
- acquire equipment to help you fight and escape fires
- devise and regularly practice an escape plan

Four Steps for Safety

Remove Potential Fire Hazards and Correct Unsafe Practices

For this step you'll begin outside the house. Keep your roof, gutters, and outside property areas of your home clean and free of debris (such as leaves and garbage) that could feed a fire. Inside and out, keep matches, lighters, candles, and other heat sources locked away out of children's sight and reach. Each year, children start many fires. About half of these fires are started with matches and lighters, so teach your children that matches are tools, not toys. Your child learns that he should never use his dad's drill, and he can learn the same rule for matches. Children as young as 2 years old are capable of lighting cigarette lighters and matches, so it's a good idea to combine teaching with keeping matches and lighters out of reach—no matter how obedient your toddler seems to be. Discard any lighters that are not child-resistant, but remember that child-resistant is not childproof.

If there is a smoker in the house, another hazard and another set of rules must be considered. Never smoke in bed or when you are drowsy. Don't leave a lit cigarette unattended in the ashtray, and always use deep, sturdy ashtrays. Make sure cigarettes are properly extinguished before emptying the ashtrays. Even cigarette butts can ignite trash. Better yet, encourage all smokers to go outside; an added benefit will be that your child will be kept away from harmful secondhand tobacco smoke.

Use caution with electronic cigarettes. Fires have occurred while e-cigarettes were being used, the battery was being charged, or the device was being transported. Battery failures have led to small explosions, some of which have resulted in serious injuries. Never leave charging e-cigarettes unattended, especially where children can reach them. Don't let batteries come in contact with coins, keys, or other metals in your pocket. Always follow the manufacturer's instructions for safe charging, use and disposal. Always keep the device away from flammable or combustible materials, such as a bed or soft furnishings. (See Chapter 10, "Common Poisons in the Home," for more information on e-cigarettes.)

Burning candles is another safety hazard that is easily addressed— avoid using them as long as small children are in your home. In addition to the special instructions found in Chapter 15, "Debra's Holiday Safety Guide," there are some general rules to follow no matter what the age of family members:

- never use candles near draperies or anything else that might easily catch fire
- do not allow children or teens to have candles in their bedrooms
- never leave candles unattended.

Candles stored for emergencies or other special needs should be locked away out of the sight and reach of children.

Anyplace where fire is used as a tool, extra precautions must be taken, and the room in which this happens most is the kitchen. You may wish to go back to Chapter 2, "Preventing Injuries in the Kitchen," to review ways to avoid burns and unwanted fires there. Anywhere in the house, if you are going to be standing or walking near a stove, fireplace, or open space heater, do not wear long, loose-fitting garments, for they are more likely to catch fire than short, fitted clothing.

DO IT YOURSELF?

**Cleaning your chimney
or fireplace . . .
Not!**
Employ a professional for
this job.

A space heater should be used with caution. Place any such unit at least 3 feet away from walls, upholstered furniture, drapes, bedding, rugs, and other combustible materials. And be sure to read and carefully follow the manufacturer's instructions regarding use of the heater. Don't leave space heaters turned on when you leave a room or go to sleep. Never leave a child or pet alone with a space heater; stay close to supervise.

Use the same kind of smart approach with your fireplace. Employ a professional chimney sweep to inspect and clean your home's chimney and fireplace annually. Unless you are trained to do this work, it should not be considered a do-it-yourself project. Maintenance is crucial, for creosote builds up in chimney flues and can cause a chimney fire. Once your fireplace has been inspected and cleaned, continue to use caution. Use a sturdy fireplace screen in front of any open flame.

Think about heat sources when you choose a place to store flammable material. All flammable liquids such as gasoline, paint thinners, and kerosene should be kept in properly labeled, tightly closed, safety-approved containers. These products should be stored out of the reach of children, outside the house in a locked shed or detached garage. Keep them in a well-ventilated place away from any source of ignition and always take the containers outside to fuel power mowers and other equipment.

In Chapter 4, "Bathroom Safety," being careful with electric appliances and cords was considered, but there are some issues left to be mentioned. It is important to inspect electric appliances and cords on a regular basis. Replace frayed extension cords and appliances that have worn or loose connections. Do not overload electrical outlets, even though some items you use will make additional plug-ins available. And do not run electrical cords under carpeting or hang them from nails or doors. Those cords should not be treated as casually as a rope or piece of twine. You could get the shock of your life—literally.

Your great-great-grandma may have had to wait for a sunny day to do the family laundry, but all that changed with the widespread use of the electric or gas clothes dryer. This common, everyday appliance can cause a fire if not properly attended. Check your dryer's exhaust duct (usually a tube that runs from the back of your dryer to a wall vent). If it's made of plastic, replace it with metal, which won't burn if lint lodges inside and catches fire. If the duct is metal but is crushed or bent, replace it. This will eliminate a place where lint could build up. Carefully follow the manufacturer's maintenance procedures and be sure to clean the lint filter after each use. Go out and remove any obstructions around the exterior vent cap, and trim shrubbery to maintain at least 12 inches of clearance. One more thing: Do not leave home or go to sleep with your dryer running unattended.

Despite all these precautions, a house might still catch on fire. Never leave young children home alone or unsupervised—not even for a few minutes. Dress your children for bed in sleepwear that is made from flame-resistant materials. Look for garments made from 100 percent polyester, which is inherently flame-resistant. Sleepwear (larger than 9 months, up to size 14) must be flame-resistant or snug-fitting to meet CPSC sleepwear requirements. Do not put children to sleep in loose-fitting T-shirts or other oversize clothing made from cotton or cotton blends. These garments can catch fire easily and burn rapidly. Loose-fitting clothes hang away from the body, which makes contact with an ignition source more likely. Loose-fitting clothing allows an air space next to the body that helps keep the fire burning.

If you choose non-flame resistant sleepwear, make sure it is snug-fitting. The term *snug-fitting* means that the garment is almost skin-tight, fitting tightly at wrists, ankles, and waist. Moreover, it should fit the child now, not be purchased in a larger size to fit later.

Install and Maintain Smoke Alarms

Smoke alarms are your family's first line of defense against fires. These devices sound a loud alarm to warn you in time to escape a fire. They can cut in half your family's risk of dying in a home fire. Many of the deaths and injuries suffered in a fire are actually caused by smoke and poisonous gases because they rise ahead of the flames. Even when you are awake, you might not see a fire until after the smoke or gas claims a life in your home.

The first thing to do, then, is purchase a smoke alarm. (Because smoke alarms are required by law in many localities, check codes and regulation requirements with your municipality or fire department before you purchase one.) Battery-operated smoke alarms can cost from $7 to $25, depending on their features, and can be purchased at your local discount or hardware store. Electrical smoke alarms with battery backup systems are excellent choices for your protection. These alarms, which can cost from $25 to $30, are hardwired into your home's

The Safe Baby

electrical system. These should be installed by a qualified electrician. Both you and the electrician should read the manufacturer's instructions. Many fire departments will come to your home and offer advice on proper installation. Some will provide smoke alarms free to families in need and many will do the installation.

Installing smoke alarms isn't the end of the matter—they must be maintained. Every single alarm in the house must be in working order. Test each one monthly, using the test button, whether battery-operated or hard-wired. Replace batteries once a year in all smoke alarms that do not have long-life batteries. An easy way to remember to change them is to do it in the spring or fall when you change the clocks for daylight saving time. If an alarm chirps between those times, change the battery then, too. Follow the manufacturer's instructions. If remembering to change a battery isn't your forte, use a smoke alarm that comes with a 10-year, nonreplaceable lithium battery. Never remove a battery from a smoke alarm to use even temporarily in another battery-operated item, such as in a child's toy. Clean the alarm regularly, following the manufacturer's instructions, to keep it dust-free. Replace the alarm every 10 years.

Acquire Equipment to Help You Fight and Escape Fires

As a general rule, firefighting should be left to the fire department. Only adults who know how to use portable fire extinguishers should use them.

Purchase multipurpose extinguishers that are listed by a qualified testing laboratory and install them in the kitchen, basement, and workshop area. Put them in plain view but out of reach of your children. Take the time to learn how to operate the equipment before an emergency strikes. Use the extinguisher only for small, confined fires. While you are extinguishing a small fire, have everyone else in the home exit, and telephone the fire department.

Consider purchasing an automatic fire sprinkler system so that a fire will be attacked in its early stages. A system like this sprays water on the area where fire is detected. Working sprinklers decrease risk of dying in a reported fire by about 80 percent, according to the nonprofit National Fire Protection Association. It is less costly to install such a system when a house is under construction, but it can also be installed in an existing home. Used in conjunction with smoke alarms, a sprinkler system is extremely effective in protecting your family from fire.

DO IT YOURSELF!

Install smoke alarms in all the right places.

- Read and carefully follow the manufacturer's instructions.
- Mount smoke alarms high on walls or ceilings because smoke rises. If a room has a pitched (slanted) ceiling, mount the unit near the ceiling's highest point, 4 to 12 inches away from the wall. If the room has an A-frame ceiling, mount the unit at least 4 to 12 inches away from the peak. Wall-mounted alarms should be installed not more than 12 inches away from the ceiling (to the top of the alarm).
- Place alarms away from air vents, windows, doors, fireplaces, or high air flow. Do not place a smoke alarm in a corner where the ceiling meets the wall.
- Avoid placing smoke alarms in kitchens or bathrooms where cooking fumes, steam, or exhaust fumes could trigger false alarms.
- Install smoke alarms in every bedroom, outside each separate sleeping area, and on every level of the home, including the basement. For the best protection, make sure all smoke alarms are interconnected—either wired or wireless. When one sounds, they all sound. Be aware of the two most commonly recognized smoke detection technologies: ionization smoke alarms and photoelectric smoke alarms. An ionization smoke alarm, in general, is more responsive to flaming fires. A photoelectric smoke alarm, in general, is more responsive to smoldering fires. Use both types of alarms or use combination alarms, which include both technologies in a single device. The National Fire Protection Administration and the U.S. Fire Administration recommend having both types installed, because you never know which type of fire might start in your home.
- Don't decorate your smoke alarms; paint or stickers may keep them from working properly.

Devise and Regularly Practice an Escape Plan

There are some drills that will help your family survive in case of a home fire. Map out at least two escape routes from every room in the house. One way out is the door; the second way out may be a window. Always keep these routes clear, and be sure windows designated as fire exits have not been painted or nailed shut. Also, see that windows or doors with security bars are equipped with quick-release devices.

Practice your escape route with all family members at least twice a year. Because a house filled with smoke can frighten and disorient family members, it is critical to have an emergency plan that everyone in the family understands. The extent to which you include your children in these discussions depends on the age and level of maturity of each individual child. A toddler will be able to comprehend a little. Your infant will just be along "for the ride," but be sure to include her during practice. As your child grows and understands more, you will need to update your family escape plan. Know when he is ready to escape without your assistance. You will need to practice with him so that he is totally familiar with this plan.

Most deadly fires occur at night, so it is a good idea to conduct one of your fire drills at night as well as one during the day. Also practice using different ways out. Sound the smoke alarm as part of each practice session to get the children used to the sound of the alarms, and to help them know what to do when they hear the sound. If you live in an apartment, become familiar with the building's evacuation plan, and in case of fire, remember to take the stairs, not the elevator. Decide in advance which parent will be responsible for helping each young child out of the house. (Note: Children and the elderly can sleep through the sound of a smoke alarm or not hear it go off when awake; a parent/ caregiver needs to be prepared to help others get out of the home.)

Designate a fixed place outside the home (a safe distance from your home)—such as a lamppost, tree or mailbox—where family members will meet. Don't make the meeting place a vehicle or any other object that can be moved.

All family members should go to the meeting place and wait until everyone is accounted for. Tell responding firefighters whether everyone is out or who needs rescue and where they might be located.

Practice is the key to a good fire safety plan. Even small children, with practice, can understand the directions in the sidebar. You'll also need to prepare your children for seeing a firefighter, helping them understand what the firefighter is there to do. Even though firefighters are seen regularly on television shows and have been lauded for their courage, seeing a firefighter up close can still be scary for a child. Explain to her that firefighters need to wear protective clothes to keep them from getting burned. They use equipment to help them breathe, protecting them against smoke inhalation. Although firefighters may look like

---

DO IT YOURSELF!

Teach your children essential fire survival skills.

- Get out fast and stay out. Do not hide in closets or under beds or in any other area inside the home. Call 911 from a neighbor's phone and never go back into the burning house for any reason! Reinforce with your child that he must not stop or return for anything, such as a toy or pet. Never go back!
- Stop, drop, cover, and roll. If your clothes catch on fire, stop; drop to the ground right where you are; cover your face with your hands; roll over and over and back and forth to smother the flames.
- Feel a door with the back of your hand before opening it. If the door is hot do not open it (use an alternate exit); if the door is cool, open it slowly and proceed with caution. Move quickly to the nearest exit.
- Get low and go under the smoke, where the air is safer to breathe.

Practice these skills!

---

aliens from another planet when they come to fight a fire, they will be there to help protect the family. Show her a picture of a firefighter in full regalia or take her to your local fire station for a tour.

If you are trapped in a burning building, close all the doors between you and the fire. Line the doors with towels or clothing (ideally, they should be damp) to keep the smoke from coming into the room. If there is a phone in the room, call 911 or the fire department. If there is no phone in the room, go to the window and signal for help by waving a bright-colored cloth or shining a flashlight.

The rules for fire safety should be applied everywhere your children visit. When your child is ready, make a game of having him apply the rules to the school, library, movie theater, and friends' homes. Make sure your child knows at least two ways to get out of any building. Teach him to be fire smart.

Review and Safety Checklist

☑ Remove potential fire hazards from your home and use caution with all flammable products.

☑ Clean debris from around your home and keep lighters and matches locked away.

☑ Properly extinguish cigarettes and never leave lit cigarettes unattended.

☑ Never leave charging e-cigarettes unattended, especially where children can reach them.

☑ Use space heaters with caution.

☑ Periodically have the fireplace cleaned by a professional.

☑ Store flammable material away from heat sources.

☑ Periodically inspect electric cords and appliances.

☑ Carefully follow the manufacturer's maintenance procedures for your dryer. Clean the lint filter after each use and never leave the house or go to sleep while it is running.

☑ Dress the children for bed in flame-resistant clothing. Do not put children to bed in loose-fitting cotton garments.

☑ Install and maintain smoke alarms.

☑ Devise and regularly practice an escape plan.

☑ Teach your children fire survival skills.

Gun Safety

Each year, approximately 50 children age 14 years and under die from an unintentional gun shooting. The best way to protect children from injury and death due to a firearm is to remove all guns from places children live and play.

Even if you do not have guns in your home, you must realize that other parents have made a different decision. This chapter is for all parents, because if your child visits a home where a gun is kept, you (and she) need to know some basic rules. Don't think it is just older children you need to protect. Children as young as 3 years old are strong enough to pull a trigger.

For Parents Who Keep Guns

If you store firearms in your home, it is your responsibility to ensure that they are not accessible to unauthorized users, especially inquisitive young children. It is recommended that you follow these safety guidelines, which all experts agree can save lives.

Store Guns Locked, Out of Reach and Out of Sight

Keep unloaded firearms in a locked gun cabinet, safe, or gun vault. Ammunition should be stored and locked away in a separate location. Keep the keys and lock combinations to these cabinets in a place where your child cannot find them.

Use a Child Safety Lock

Children have been known to find firearms that are "hidden," so an additional safety precaution should be followed for extra protection:

Use cable-style gun locks if this type fits your firearm; otherwise, use another approved gun-locking device, such as a trigger lock. Install such devices on your unloaded firearms, being careful to follow the directions that come with the device. Be sure to get your safety product from a reputable company. Never install a gun lock on a loaded gun; even with the lock in place, the firearm could discharge.

Incidentally, air guns, BB guns, pellet guns, and paint guns should also be kept out of children's hands. Thousands of children aged 14 and under are treated in hospital emergency rooms annually for nonpowder, gun-related injuries.

For Parents Who Don't Own a Gun . . . As Well As Parents Who Do
Ask Your Friends and Relatives

Studies show that more than 40 percent of households in the United States have a firearm in them. There's nothing wrong with asking the parents of your relatives and your children's friends—or anyone else whom your children may visit—if they own firearms and are practicing safe storage methods. Based on their answers, you can make the choice whether to allow your children to visit there.

Teach Your Child

Every child from preschooler to teen should be taught that firearms can hurt and kill people. Teach them this rule: If you see a gun, don't touch it; get away and tell an adult. In addition, tell them to follow the same rule if they see any other kind of weapon or dangerous instrument, such as a syringe.

Teach your young child the difference between a toy gun and a real one. Before age 8, few children can reliably distinguish what's real from what's not. Children watching TV and movies and seeing people firing guns may not fully understand that the people they are watching are just actors. Help your child understand that in real life, firing a gun at someone is dangerous and could kill.

Other Security Options
Home Security Options

If you wish to provide more security for your family in the face of violence in our society, there are options other than firearms to consider.

Invest in a home alarm system. Have solid-core doors for all entry points to your home and equip them with good-quality deadbolt locks. Use motion sensor lights or cameras near or around entry points. Install a peephole in your front door and always use it before opening the door. Be sure to thoroughly check references of people who work in your home. You can also organize or become involved in a neighborhood watch program. When your youngest child is at least 5 years old, consider getting a dog whose bark can scare away intruders. Consult a veterinarian regarding the best dog for your family.

Review and Safety Checklist

If you have guns in your home:

- ☑ Keep them locked in a gun cabinet or safe.
- ☑ Store your firearms and ammunition in separate locations.
- ☑ Keep both firearms and ammunition locked out of reach and out of sight of your children.
- ☑ Install gun locks or other safety devices to prevent unauthorized use of your guns.

Whether or not you keep a gun in your home:

- ☑ At homes where your child visits, ask the adults there if they have guns. Make sure everyone who has guns follows the guidelines above. If they do not, you should keep your child away.
- ☑ Teach your child the difference between toy guns and real guns.
- ☑ Teach your child this three-part rule: If you find a gun, don't touch it; get away; tell an adult.

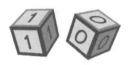

Common Poisons in the Home

Toddlers are particularly prone to unintended poisoning. They are curious, they move fast, and they explore everything with their mouths! Nearly half of the 2 million poisonings reported to poison centers across the nation each year involve children under 6 years of age who are exposed to potentially poisonous medicines and household chemicals. The best way to keep your child from ingesting poison is to keep all potentially harmful products out of sight and out of reach, in cabinets that have locks or child-resistant safety latches. Bear in mind that a child can figure out ways to get to the tallest shelves. Keeping intriguing articles out of sight is an important safety component. Taking these precautions may become second nature to you in your own home, but your awareness of such possibilities is important in homes you visit, too. Studies show that 30 percent of pediatric poisonings occur due to children's ingestion of their grandparents' medications.

It is ironic that products we bring into the house to help our children can be toxic to them. While medicine created especially for children may not be considered a poison by most folks, the wrong dosage can kill. (This is true, as well, for adults.) When giving medicine to your child, don't just read the label and decide it's the right thing for a specific situation. Check with the pediatrician first. Once you have her approval, carefully follow directions on the label—dosage is likely to be based on weight and age—and use the measuring dispenser that comes packaged with the medication.

Another way we may bring in toxic substances is by wearing them on our clothes. Family members who work with poisonous materials should shower, if possible, and change clothes and shoes before leaving work. This reduces the possibility of toxins from the workplace being carried into your car or home.

Poisonous Products in the House
Guard Against Mistaken Identity
Teach your children to always ask permission before eating or drinking anything, and store harmful products away from food. Never put harmful products side by side with food and keep all products in their original containers. Any family member might ingest something that you have transferred to a milk jug, jar, or 2-liter bottle, mistaking the contents for something meant to be consumed. Moreover, labels on original containers will assist medical caregivers or personnel at poison control centers in the event of a poisoning.

The same rules apply to medicines, vitamins, and supplements. Something that is good for adults may be poisonous for children. For example, although iron supplements are safe for adults who follow label instructions, ingestion of only a few of them can be lethal to young children, depending on the amount of iron per tablet and the weight of the child. Simply putting these items on a high shelf in the kitchen or in the bathroom medicine cabinet is not safe. Keep all medicines—both prescription and over-the-counter—as well as vitamins and supplements in a locked cabinet out of the reach of children. If you keep medications or any other potentially harmful products in your handbag, don't leave it within reach of any child. Remember this precaution when you visit a home that has children or when you have visitors in your home. If Aunt Polly comes to visit and puts her purse on the floor beside her chair, cheerfully tell her you are putting her purse in the same place you keep yours, which is out of the sight and reach of children.

After you have used any medication—even supplements or vitamins—securely close the child-resistant cap and promptly return the bottle to its place. Once again the mantra: child-resistant does not mean childproof! Remember to never call medicine *candy.* In addition, because young ones tend to imitate adults, avoid taking medicines in front of children.

Keep All Cleaning Products Out of Your Child's Sight and Reach

Like medicine, there are poisonous products that are good when used as intended. Just as we take precautions with fire, we must take care with poisonous products. Many household cleaning products are toxic. Using these products incorrectly endangers the health of your family and the air quality in your home. Improper storage may lead to unintentional poisoning. Improper disposal can pollute our drinking water.

Start by being careful from the very beginning—in the store. Buy plant-based and water-based products when possible. Select the least toxic product you can find and completely avoid purchasing products labeled *Danger* or *Poison;* typically they are the most hazardous.

The EPA has a list of products that meet its Safer Choice requirements for cleaning and other needs. They include cleaning products for home and vehicles; the website is *epa.gov/safer-choice*. For a product to carry the Safer Choice logo, all its ingredients must pass the program's health and environment criteria. It must also meet requirements around packaging, performance and ingredient disclosure.

Fragrances can irritate eyes or lungs, so look for labels stating "Fragrance Free." Unlike products advertised as "unscented," which contain masking fragrances to hide the chemical smell, these products are what they claim to be—fragrance-free.

When you must buy products containing hazardous substances, buy only the amount you expect to use, and use it as soon as possible.

Before using the product, make sure you read the labels and follow those directions carefully. Wear protective equipment, such as gloves, as recommended by the manufacturer. Never mix cleaning products or chemicals unless directions indicate you can safely do so, especially ammonia and bleach, which together produce a toxic gas. Use products in a well-ventilated place; open windows and use a fan to circulate the air toward the outside, and keep children away from the area. Securely close the product lid as soon as the product is used. Do not re-use empty household cleaning product containers. Store all cleaning products—even less toxic ones—in a locked cabinet or cabinet secured with child-resistant safety latches.

Practice preventive measures. When there is a spill, clean it up as soon as possible, before it has time to set, thus cutting down the amount of cleaner needed. Before using so-called air fresheners that simply cover odors, try airing out the house. Use liners to catch spills. Protect yourself, too, by not smoking or eating while using poisonous products.

Even in safe homes where products are carefully stored, poisoning can occur when the product is taken out of storage and is in use. Therefore be extra cautious when using harmful products around children.

Make Your Own Cleaning Products

The most toxic household products are corrosive or caustic cleaners. They contain lye or acids, and they are found in drain cleaners, oven cleaners, and toilet-bowl cleaners. They are the most dangerous cleaning products to have around the house because they can burn skin, eyes, and internal tissue at the slightest contact. Using homemade products is a tradition in my family, passed from my grandmother to my mother to me. Here are some do-it-yourself alternatives to highly toxic products:

INSTEAD OF	USE
Drain cleaner	A plunger or plumber's snake.
Oven cleaner	Steel wool and baking soda; add salt for tough stains. (Not recommended for continuous- cleaning ovens and self-cleaning ovens.)
Toilet bowl cleaner	Toilet brush and baking soda or vinegar. (This will not disinfect.)
Glass cleaner	1 Tbsp. vinegar in 1 qt. water. Spray on and use newspaper to wipe dry.
Furniture polish	1 tsp. lemon juice in 1 pt. vegetable oil. Wipe on, then off.
All-purpose cleaner	4 Tbsp. baking soda in 1 qt. warm water. Apply with a cloth (or paper towel if meat, poultry, seafood juices are present) and rinse with clear water.

Use only recipes obtained from reputable sources, and don't concoct your own brews. If you have any questions about mixing products together, call the product manufacturers to find out if they recommend the mixture or if there are hazards associated with using their products in ways not specifically stated on the label. Safe storage is required even with homemade products, and they must be labeled. Note the exact ingredients and the purpose for the product. You think you'll remember, but in a month or two—trust me!—you will not recall what is in that unlabeled container. When choosing a container, never put your homemade products in a milk jug, cup, or 2-liter bottle.

Be Aware of Dead Ringers (Look-Alike Products)

Some poisonous products look exactly like foods and drinks our children commonly ingest. Even an older child or an adult can easily make a mistake and unintentionally ingest such products, so take special care to securely store them away after use. Some examples are chocolate laxatives that look like candy bars, pills that look like candy, clear lamp oil that looks like bottled water, and colored lamp oil that looks like mouthwash.

Laundry Products

Keep Single-load Laundry Packets Away from Children

Children often mistake those squishy, brightly colored liquid laundry packets/pods for candy, toys, or teething rings. These enticing-looking, bite-size packets are filled with highly concentrated, toxic chemicals. Each year, nearly 12,000 children, ages 5 and under, are harmed by laundry packets, according to the American Association of Poison Control Centers. Unfortunately, since 2012, there have been eight reported deaths in the U.S. associated with laundry pack exposure. Two were young children, but six of those fatalities were adults with dementia.

It can take just a few seconds for a child to swallow the toxic chemicals or to get the chemicals in their eyes. As with all cleaning products, *do not* let children handle laundry packets. Keep the packets sealed in their original packaging, and make sure they are locked up high and out of a child's sight and reach after every use. If a packet is swallowed or its contents get into the eye, immediately call Poison Help at 800-222-1222.

I strongly recommend not using the packets if your home has children under 6 years of age, or if anyone in your household is cognitively impaired. Instead, use traditional liquid or powder detergents (in the bottle or box); these are much less concentrated than laundry packets.

Batteries
Keep Button Batteries Out of Sight

Button batteries are small and shiny. When swallowed, a coin-sized lithium battery can lodge in the throat of a child. Saliva triggers an electrical current, causing a chemical reaction that can severely burn the esophagus in as little as two hours. The chemicals in the batteries can also cause serious harm to a child if the battery is inserted into the ear or nose. According to Safe Kids Worldwide, each year in the United States, more than 2,800 kids are treated in emergency rooms after swallowing button batteries. In some cases, children have died from their injuries.

Lithium batteries can be found in many household items, such as remote controls, toys, singing greeting cards, digital thermometers, flameless candles, calculators, key fobs, watches, and flashing holiday jewelry or decorations. Know which items and devices in your home have button batteries. Children love to pick up gadgets, play with them and take them apart. Duct tape battery compartments if they do not have a screw to secure them closed, and keep these objects out of the sight and reach of small children. Store any loose batteries in a locked cabinet. Don't insert or change batteries in front of small children. Moreover, "dead" batteries almost always contain enough life to generate an electrical current once ingested, so, it's important to dispose of them immediately and safely. Closely supervise children who are playing with devices that are powered by button batteries.

The National Battery Ingestion Hotline (run by the National Capital Poison Center) advises: If you suspect your child has ingested a battery or put one in his nose or ear, go to the nearest emergency room immediately. Complications are delayed, so even an asymptomatic child is at risk. Call the Battery Hotline at 800-498-8666 (or 202-625-3333). If the battery was swallowed, don't let the child eat or drink until an x-ray shows the battery is beyond the esophagus.

Liquid Nicotine
Keep Children Away from E-Cigarettes

Most of the liquid nicotine sold for e-cigarettes is bright and colorful and comes in a variety of sweet-smelling flavors children find appealing. Liquid nicotine is highly concentrated, and even a small amount is poisonous. Less than half a teaspoon can be fatal to a toddler, warns the American Academy of Pediatrics. Poisonings can also occur when liquid nicotine is inhaled or absorbed through the skin or eyes.

A study published in the journal *Pediatrics* found that from January 2012 to April 2015, the monthly number of child exposures to e-cigarettes increased by about 1,500%. As more people began using e-cigarettes, the rate of childhood exposures rose drastically. The Child Nicotine Poisoning Prevention Act, signed into law in 2016, requires child resistant packaging on liquid nicotine containers.

Make certain all e-cigarettes, e-nicotine refills and cartridges are locked up and stored out of your child's sight and reach.

I strongly recommend that you *not* use or store e-cigarettes, liquid nicotine, and related products in the home. However, if you or someone else in your home must use them, here are some guidelines:

- Use and refill alone, because children imitate adults. Using e-cigarettes and refilling them while children are nearby could lead to dangerous exposure.
- Follow the specific disposal instructions on the label to safely dispose of e-cigarettes and their parts. Vapes are easy to pull apart, and their small parts present a choking hazard.
- Be aware of guests who may come to your home with e-cigarettes in their purse, briefcase or backpack. Make sure the devices are properly stored out of children's sight and reach.
- If you think someone has been exposed to an e-cigarette or liquid nicotine, call the Poison Help line immediately.

(See Chapter 11, "Environmental Hazards," for more information on e-cigarettes.)

Alcohol
Keep Alcohol Away from Children
Children are much more sensitive than adults to the toxic effects of alcohol. Alcohol can cause a child's blood sugar to plunge to a dangerously low level, which can lead to seizures, coma, and even death in a young child. In addition, keep out of the reach of your children any alcohol-laced products, such as:

- mouthwash (read the label—the alcohol content of these products varies significantly with different brands)
- perfume, cologne, or aftershave
- vanilla extract and lemon extract
- cough/cold medications
- rubbing alcohol
- antifreeze and windshield-washer fluid

Most hand sanitizers contain 60-65% ethyl alcohol, also known as ethanol. This is the same type of alcohol found in beer (3-6% alcohol) and spirits (40% alcohol). Any of these can be hazardous to children. While a lick or taste of hand sanitizer should not be enough to be toxic, as little as a teaspoon of it could intoxicate a toddler. To make it less likely for your child to be tempted to try a taste, avoid buying scented hand sanitizers, particularly those with fruity scents. If you carry a small container of hand sanitizer in your purse, you have one more reason not to put your purse down within reach of any child. Do not leave this product on a table or counter or any place else where a child might grab it. When not in use, hand sanitizers should be kept in a secure location, a locked cabinet. You know why: because everything goes in the mouth.

Poisonous Plants
Recognize Which Plants Are Poisonous
Some of the plants that are used to beautify your house and yard may be toxic, so it's important to identify all the different plants both in and around your home. Because several different plants may have the same common name, find out both the botanical and common name. A list of common poisonous plants can be found in Appendix B.

Obtain from the poison center or your local cooperative extension agent a list of the common poisonous plants that grow in your area. You can also take the plant or a cutting to a reputable and experienced nursery, florist, or plant store for identification. Make a list or put a label on every plant, so in case of ingestion you will have pertinent information available. Be sure your family can identify dangerous plants such as poison oak, ivy and sumac. If someone touches one of these plants, rinse the skin that touched the plant right away with soap and running water for at least 5 minutes.

Your child, attracted to a plant's color or shape, may put parts of it in her mouth, perhaps swallowing it. Symptoms that may occur when this happens include:

- skin, eye, and mouth irritation
- breathing problems
- allergic reactions
- stomach or other pain
- vomiting and diarrhea

Use Only Nontoxic Plants During Your Child's Early Years

I recommend that you purchase only nontoxic plants when you have pets or children under the age of 6. Toxic plants outside the home should either be removed or fenced in. Inside the home, hang plants from the ceiling. (Choose lightweight pots and secure them with a closed fastening device.) But still keep an eye out for fallen leaves. Even in the case of nontoxic plants, a child may ingest soil, which may contain pesticides or fertilizer. Further, a child can choke on any leaf, even a nontoxic one.

If Aunt Polly brings a plant with her as a gift, ask her what it is. Ignore her raised eyebrows when you tell her you like to label all your plants. "Aunt Polly, this is so lovely. I want to hang it from the ceiling where everyone can admire it. Yes, Aunt Polly, it may be hard to water it up there, but I don't mind at all!"

Reinforce with your children the rule that they should not eat or put into their mouths any leaves, stems, flowers, twigs, wild berries, mushrooms, or any parts of shrubs or garden or ornamental plants. Keep an eagle eye on your child after rainy weather, when wild mushrooms are abundant.

First Aid Tips and Emergency Measures

Be Ready to Reach Poison Control Quickly

Remember this telephone number: 1-800-222-1222. It's the toll-free Poison Help line. Call it from anywhere in the U.S., day or night, seven days a week. You will be connected automatically to a specially trained nurse or pharmacist at your local poison center. Post this number on the refrigerator and program it into your cell phone and home phone. (Call now for free phone stickers and refrigerator magnets.)

If you prefer to get expert help online, use webPOISONCONTROL®, a new web tool and app that helps you manage a poisoning by providing case-specific triage and home treatment recommendations. webPOISONCONTROL was created by poison centers and is maintained by board certified medical and clinical toxicologists, so you know it is safe and reliable information that you can trust. To try it out, go to *triage.webpoisoncontrol.org* and find out what to do at home, or if you should go to the emergency room or get additional help from your local poison center. webPOISONCONTROL is also available as a free app from Google Play or the App Store that can be downloaded to your mobile device.

Your best bet is to always call the poison center before calling your doctor because you are more likely to talk to an expert right away at the Poison Help line. You may need to wait for a call back from your doctor. However, if the situation appears life threatening (for example, if your child is choking, collapsed, or having trouble breathing), call 911. In all other cases, calling poison control will enable you to speak to a specialist who can assess the severity of the situation. The call is confidential.

Prioritize Your Actions When You Suspect Poisoning

1. Check your child's mouth and carefully remove any remaining poison. You may need to wipe out her mouth with a damp washcloth.
2. Call the Poison Help Line before administering anything by mouth. Call as soon as you suspect a poisoning; do not wait until symptoms are displayed.
3. Bring the ingested product (or its container) to the telephone when you call the Poison Help line and take it with you if you

must visit the emergency room or doctor's office. If a poisonous plant is the cause, refer to the label you made or the list you keep and take the information with you.

Important: Do not induce vomiting—doing so often makes the situation worse. When you call the Poison Help line, you will talk to a specialist who can tell you the correct treatment to administer. The American Academy of Pediatrics now recommends that syrup of ipecac no longer be used routinely as a home treatment and that parents should safely dispose of the syrup of ipecac currently in their homes.

If poison gets into the eye:
1. Flood the eye with lukewarm (never hot) water. Pour the water from a large glass or pitcher held 2 or 3 inches from the eye. Let the water hit the bridge of the nose and gently run into the eyes rather than pouring the water directly into the eye. You don't have to hold the eye open, but have your child blink under the stream of water as much as possible. Continue for at least 15 minutes.
2. Call the Poison Help line or visit *triage.webpoisoncontrol.org.*

If poison gets on the skin:
1. Remove any contaminated clothing and flood skin with water for 15 minutes.
2. Wash gently with soap and water, then rinse.
3. Call the Poison Help line or visit *triage.webpoisoncontrol.org.*

If poison is inhaled:
1. Immediately move to fresh air.
2. Call 911 if the victim appears short of breath.
3. Open doors and windows wide.
4. Call the Poison Help line or visit *triage.webpoisoncontrol.org.*

Poison Patrol Checklist: What to Look For
In the house and yard:
- ☑ tobacco and e-cigarette products, especially liquid nicotine
- ☑ plants and plant food
- ☑ button batteries (such as found in key fobs and remote controls)
- ☑ broken plaster

☑ paint chips and painted toys (may contain lead—see next chapter for details)

In the kitchen:

☑ window and counter cleaners
☑ dishwasher products, detergents, soaps, oven cleaners
☑ drain cleaners
☑ ammonia
☑ cleanser and scouring powder
☑ carpet and upholstery cleaner
☑ furniture polish
☑ pet products such as flea and tick collars and powders
☑ vitamins, supplements (natural or herbal), and medications, including aspirin

On the table:

☑ green or sprouted potatoes (they contain a toxin called solanine, which can cause gastrointestinal problems)
☑ table salt (as little as half a teaspoon for an infant or a tablespoon for a toddler can cause damage to the central nervous system)

In the bathroom:

☑ cosmetics
☑ all grooming products
☑ baby powder and baby oil
☑ shampoos and conditioners
☑ hair straighteners and relaxers
☑ hair dyes
☑ hair removers
☑ creams
☑ nail polish and polish remover
☑ deodorants
☑ perfumes, colognes, aftershaves
☑ hand sanitizers
☑ contact lens disinfectants
☑ insect repellents
☑ arthritis pain relief ointment
☑ Visine eye drops
☑ suntan lotions

☑ mouthwash

☑ fluoride toothpaste (ingesting large amounts—most or all of the tube—may cause symptoms of fluoride toxicity; use a pea-size amount of toothpaste for children under 6)

☑ medications, both prescription and over-the-counter, including aspirin, vitamins, natural or herbal supplements, and iron pills

☑ rubbing alcohol

☑ jewelry cleaner

☑ toilet bowl cleaners

☑ disinfectants

☑ room deodorizer

In the garage, basement, and storage areas:

☑ pest control products

☑ weed killers and fertilizers

☑ gasoline and car-care products such as antifreeze (*see note below), motor oil, brake fluid, and windshield-washer solution

☑ turpentine, paints, and paint thinner

☑ pool supplies

☑ kerosene

☑ art and hobby supplies

☑ glues and adhesives

☑ charcoal lighters

Note: The main ingredient in many major antifreeze brands is ethylene glycol, which is very toxic. In the past, this antifreeze had a sweet taste that enticed children and pets to drink large amounts of it if it was left out in open containers or if it had spilled in the garage or on the driveway. In December 2012, all U.S. antifreeze manufacturers voluntarily agreed to add a bittering agent to antifreeze. But bittering agents have never been shown to be effective in actual pediatric poisonings, so be careful to protect children and pets from ingesting antifreeze. Use antifreeze formulated with propylene glycol, which is considerably less toxic.

In the laundry room:

☑ soaps and detergents

☑ laundry packets/pods

☑ bleach

☑ fabric softeners

☑ stain remover

In closets:

☑ moth balls
☑ shoe polish

In bedrooms:

☑ pain relievers and other medicines
☑ perfumes and colognes
☑ room fresheners
☑ hearing aid or remote control batteries

In handbags:

☑ cosmetics
☑ pain relievers and other medicines
☑ hand sanitizers
☑ cigarettes or other nicotine products

Make sure poison prevention precautions are taken in all the places your baby frequently visits, such as the homes of grandparents, other relatives, and friends.

Review and Safety Checklist

So that you won't mistake one product for another, leave all products in their original, labeled containers. Even with those labels, you should never store harmful products in a refrigerator or pantry.

☑ Read labels carefully. Select the least toxic product you can find whenever possible and always try to buy plant-based or water-based products.

☑ When using toxic substances, keep children away. Protect yourself, too, by not smoking or eating when using any kinds of toxins.

☑ Remember: Out of reach and out of sight for all medicines, cleaning products, alcohol, and other harmful products. Keep them locked away from young children at all times.

☑ Follow recipes from reputable sources when making your own cleaning products and carefully note all ingredients and the purpose of the concoction. You're making these products for safety's sake, but they can be toxic if ingested or handled improperly.

☑ As long as you have pets or have children under the age of 6 in your home, use only nontoxic plants.

☑ Post the Poison Help line number—1-800-222-1222—on the refrigerator, and program it into your cell phone and home phone.

☑ Prioritize your actions when you suspect poisoning.

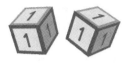

Environmental Hazards

You cannot always depend on your nose and eyes to tell you when something is poisonous. Four toxins examined in this chapter—lead, arsenic, radon, and carbon monoxide—are invisible and odorless. Another, secondhand smoke, is a toxin that can be seen and smelled—by nonsmokers. As any reformed smoker knows, the odor of cigarette smoke clinging to skin, clothing, and fabric in the home can be nauseating. However, the dangers secondhand smoke poses, especially for children, go far beyond that kind of discomfort. Another class of poison, pesticide, is brought into the home deliberately when it is deemed necessary to eliminate harmful pests. As we consider these products, we shall weigh their benefits against the potential harm they introduce. And we'll discuss some less toxic methods for ridding the home of harmful pests. Finally we'll go back into the nursery, this time to consider what harmful chemicals may lurk there and what to do about them.

Lead

The brains and nervous systems of young children are quite sensitive to the damaging effects of lead. Indeed, because lead is more easily absorbed into the growing bodies of fetuses, infants, and children, they are more vulnerable to lead exposure than adults. This danger has not gone away. Lead continues to be a serious health risk for children, even though the CPSC banned the use of lead-based paint for residential use in 1978. The reason is simple: lead is a hazard that still coats the walls of millions of homes. Once disturbed it can create a fine dust, which is dangerous for children as well as adults. Children with dangerous

YOUR CHILD IS AT RISK FOR LEAD POISONING IF . . .

- Your home was built before 1978 or your child frequently visits a home or building constructed before 1978, if that building was recently remodeled or has peeling or chipping paint.
- You or any other adult living in your home works with lead.

If you believe your child has been exposed to lead, speak with your pediatrician or health department. A blood test can detect levels of lead in your child's body.

levels of lead in their blood may appear healthy. Because lead can pass through a woman's body to a fetus, pregnant women should limit their exposure to lead.

High levels of lead can cause seizures, coma, or death. Exposure to low levels of lead can harm a child's brain, nervous system, blood cells, and kidneys, which in turn can cause learning disabilities, slow development, hearing impairment, and ADHD. Since most children do not display any symptoms, the only way to know for sure if they have elevated lead levels in the blood is to have them tested.

The primary sources of lead poisoning in children today are lead-based paint and lead-contaminated dust. Lead-based paint is usually not a hazard if it is in good condition. However, problems occur when the paint peels or flakes off into chips or lead dust. The same kind of danger occurs when remodeling, renovation, or repainting is performed improperly, without safeguards to control lead dust. Your child doesn't have to eat paint chips to be poisoned. If she touches lead-contaminated dust, then puts her hands in her mouth, the lead will enter her system. Limiting your child's exposure is the best defense. If you suspect your home has lead paint, there are steps you can take to reduce the risk.

Watch Out for Peeling Paint and Wash It Away

- Keep an eye out for peeling paint or water leaks. Water leaks and moisture are the main cause of peeling paint. Sticking doors and windows can also damage paint.
- Make sure the peeling paint is promptly and safely repaired by someone trained in lead-safe work practices.
- Wash your baby's hands and face before meals, naptime, and bedtime. Teach and reinforce this washing practice with older children, too. Hands contaminated with lead dust are as sure as clean hands to go into the mouth.

- In addition to washing bottles and pacifiers each time they fall on the floor, wash toys and stuffed animals, too.
- Regularly wash floors and high wear-and-tear areas such as window frames, window sills, doors, and door frames, and anywhere your child plays. Vacuum first using a High Efficiency Particulate Air (HEPA) vacuum. Change the bag and filter according to the manufacturer's instructions. Contact your local health department—some have a HEPA vacuum loan program. Then use a wet mop with a mild detergent to get all the paint chips and lead dust. Hint: Use two mop buckets—one for soapy water and one for rinsing. Change the rinse water often.

> **DO IT YOURSELF?**
>
> **Removing lead . . . Not!**
> Leave it to professionals.

If Your Home Was Built Before 1978, Get Your Home Professionally Tested

This is especially important if you plan to remodel or renovate. Many consumers find spot kits helpful as an initial screen for the presence of lead, but while the kits give instant results via changes in color, they are not as reliable as laboratory tests. Two types of professional testing are lead inspection and lead-risk assessment. An inspection discloses the lead content of every surface in your home, but it does not reveal either the level of danger or how you should proceed. An assessment tells you if lead is present and makes recommendations for how the lead can be controlled.

If Lead Must Be Removed, Don't Do It Yourself

Removing lead is best left to professionals. Do not attempt to remove lead paint yourself. Hire a certified lead-abatement contractor. You are risking your own health if you remove lead improperly, and you may spread even more lead dust around your home. Make sure your family and your belongings are protected from lead dust. Plan to move out if the project is major or if it generates lots of dust.

Check the Soil in Your Yard and Take Appropriate Measures to Keep Lead Out

Exterior lead paint may have contaminated soil close to the house. Also, if your home is near a road that has seen a lot of traffic (and, thus, exhaust fumes) over the years, your soil may be contaminated from past use of leaded gasoline. Here's what to do if your soil is tainted with lead:

- Cover lead-tainted soil with grass sod, pine bark mulch or gravel, or plant bushes.
- Encourage your child to play in grassy areas that are lead-free.
- Have everyone remove their shoes before entering the house.
- Make sure you wash your child's hands after he has played outdoors and teach him not to eat dirt.
- Don't plant a home garden or serve food that has been grown in lead-laced soil.

Have the Water Tested

Testing your water does not have to be expensive; you can get mail-in kits from environmental laboratories for under $20. (See "Tap Water Safety" in Chapter 3, "More about the Kitchen.") Lead enters drinking water primarily through plumbing materials. Homes built before 1988 are more likely to have lead pipes, fixtures and solder. However, newer homes are also at risk; even legally "lead-free" plumbing may contain up to 8 percent lead. The most common problem is with brass or chrome-plated brass faucets and fixtures, which can leach significant amounts of lead into the water, especially hot water. To find out more about testing, call your local health department or the EPA's hotline. (See Appendix E, "Helpful Resources.")

Stick to Cold Water for Drinking and Cooking

The longer water sits in your pipes, the higher the risk for lead. Use only cold water for drinking, cooking, or preparing baby formula, because hot water is likely to contain higher levels of lead. Run the cold water for 30 to 60 seconds before catching it in a glass, cup, or pan, and if it has been more than 6 hours since you used the tap, allow the cold water to run until it becomes as cold as it will get, which may take up to 2 minutes or more. Once you have flushed your tap, you can store the cold water in your refrigerator for later use.

If you are concerned about wasting water, catch it in a container and use it for watering your plants or washing clothes. Be sure to clean faucet screens regularly, taking out any solder particles caught by the screens. If there is a high level of lead in your pipes, you may wish to

> ## PROPOSITION 65—STANDARDS FOR LEAD
>
> When shopping for dishes, look for lead-free dishes or lead-safe dishes—in other words, those that meet California's Proposition 65. Most tableware in common use does not pose a lead hazard. However, if the amount of lead that can leach into food from your dishes is greater than Proposition 65 levels, your dishes may pose a health risk. Ask the retailer or manufacturer if their product meets those standards.

purchase a filter certified for lead removal or switch to a bottled water that is known to be safe for drinking and cooking.

Know What Other Products in Your Home May Contain Lead

Glazes for some dishes and mugs contain lead. Be especially careful when purchasing items abroad. If you have a lead-glazed, ceramic container, don't heat, microwave, or serve hot food or drinks in it and don't store acidic foods (such as fruit juices) in it. That lead crystal bottle someone gave your baby is just for show; don't feed your baby with it! Any dish that is meant to be decorative should be just that—don't serve food on it. Silver-plated items or plates made from pewter, brass, or bronze should never be used for serving food to children.

In addition, lead has been found in inexpensive children's jewelry and some costume jewelry designed for adults. It is important to make sure children don't handle or mouth any jewelry.

Because metal keys have been identified as potential sources of lead exposure, babies should not be allowed to play with or chew on keys.

Remember to keep up-to-date with recalled products. Please refer to Appendix D, "Recall Information."

Check Lead Hazards in Other Environments

Child care centers and homes of family or friends that are visited often can also pose a lead hazard. If such homes or buildings were built before 1978, make sure the paint is in good condition. Also, many older school, park, and community playgrounds were painted with lead paint. Ask when the playgrounds were built and look for any signs of chipping paint or dust.

Arsenic

Check Pressure-Treated Wood in and Around Your Home

Arsenic? You may be certain there is no arsenic in your home environment, but think again. Arsenic was once a common ingredient in pressure-treated wood, in the form of chromium copper arsenate (CCA), so it may be in your deck, porch, picnic table, or play set. Arsenic is a known cancer-causing chemical. Long-term exposure to elevated levels of arsenic has been linked to skin, bladder, and lung cancer. Studies show that arsenic can be picked up from the surface of CCA-treated wood. Young children who play on or under structures made of CCA-treated wood and who put their hands in their mouths are at increased risk of exposure. Arsenic-containing residue from the wood can rub off on children's hands while they are at play and be ingested when their hands come into contact with their mouths. Thanks to a 2002 agreement between the EPA and the playground-building industry, wood treated with CCA was phased out as of December 31, 2003. If you have items in your yard that were bought prior to that date, your child may be at risk.

If your child has contact with CCA-treated wood, immediately wash his hands thoroughly with soap and water, especially before eating. The sidebar explains what you can do to protect your child.

Radon

Radon is an invisible and odorless gas that occurs naturally from the breakdown of uranium. It can be found in soil, rock, and air. When breathed outdoors, this gas poses a minimal health risk, but when it becomes trapped in buildings, concentrations build up, which can be cause for concern. If the radioactive decay products of radon get released into your lungs, they can damage the live cells lining the lungs. Years of this damage can lead to lung cancer. In the United States radon is a leading cause of lung cancer, second only to cigarette smoking.

How a home was built and what construction materials were used can affect radon levels. Local geology is another contributing factor. Every state has pockets of high radon levels. Because radon levels vary from one area to another, the only way to know a specific home's radon level is to test it. Any home can have a radon problem, no matter its age or condition and no matter whether there is a basement. Basements and first floors are more likely to have the highest radon levels. It is also

DO IT YOURSELF!

What to do about arsenic . . .
- Find it. Some CCA has a green tint, but testing is the only way to know for certain. Contact your local or state health department for more information on testing. (You may be able to contact the structure's manufacturer or builder to determine if it contains CCA-treated wood.)
- Seal it. Use a penetrating deck treatment.
- Replace it. High-exposure areas, such as handrails and steps, should be replaced with nonarsenic-containing products.
- Avoid it. Keep children and pets away from the soil and spaces beneath and around it, and do not store toys or tools there. Rain will cause the arsenic to leach onto anything beneath the treated product.
- Cover it. An arsenic-treated picnic table should be covered with a tablecloth. Do not eat, drink, or prepare food on CCA-treated surfaces.
- Don't pressure-wash it, and don't use commercial deck-washing products, which can make the arsenic even more toxic. Use soap and water instead, with cleaning tools and rags you can throw away.
- Don't let your child play on any rough wood surface treated with arsenic; the splinters are poison.

possible for your home to have an elevated radon level while a neighboring home does not.

Radon can enter your home through openings around water pipes, gas pipes, sump pumps, and drains. It can also enter through cracks and holes in the walls and foundation. The water supply is another possibility. (See item 2 below.)

According to the EPA, your family's risk of getting lung cancer from radon depends mostly on how much radon is in your home, the amount of time you spend in your home, and whether you are a smoker or have ever smoked. Smoking combined with radon is an especially serious health risk.

Test the Air in Your Home
Because of the serious health threat posed by radon, the Environmental Protection Agency recommends that all homes and apartments below

---

DO IT YOURSELF!

Testing for Radon
- Test Kits are either short-or long-term.
- Short Term Kit: 2 to 90 days. (Usually 2-10 days, though there is technology to do 11-90 day tests.) The most common is an activated charcoal canister.
- Long Term Kit: 91 days to a year. The most common is an alpha track detector.

Note: As radon levels tend to vary from day to day and season to season, a short-term test is less likely than a long-term test to tell you your year-round average radon level.

The EPA recommends that for homes, initial measurements be short-term tests placed in the lowest lived-in level. Short-term testing under closed-building conditions helps to ensure that residents quickly learn if a home contains very high levels of radon.

---

the third floor be tested. Fortunately, testing is easy and inexpensive. Your local health department may offer free kits or kits at a reduced price. Low-cost radon test kits can also be ordered from the National Radon Program Services by going to their website, *www.sosradon.org* or by calling 1-800-SOS-RADON (1-800-767-7236). You can also purchase kits at your local hardware or home improvement store. The price range is $10 to $45. You can perform your own test or you can hire a radon tester in your area who is state certified or proficient with a privately-run national radon program. Your state radon office can supply you with a list of testing kit companies and radon testers.

Insist that your child's school or child care center be tested. Some states or counties require this.

Note: Radon is measured in picoCuries per liter of air—pCi/L. Although the EPA says there is no known safe level of radon and that any radon exposure carries some risk, it has set 4pCi/L as the level at which it recommends action to reduce your home's radon level.

If the Air in Your Home Has Radon, Test the Water

If you have tested the air in your home and found a significantly high radon problem, it may be a good idea to test the water, also, as a possible source of radon entry. If you are on a public water supply, call the utility company for more information. If your water comes from a private well, contact a lab that is certified to measure radiation to test your water—especially if you live in an area that is known to have high levels of radon in water.

Be Aware That There Are a Variety of Ways to Lower Radon Levels

Don't despair if testing indicates elevated levels of radon in your home. There are a variety of ways to lower radon levels. Radon-reduction techniques—preventing the entry of radon or removing radon and its decay products from the air in your home—should be performed only by a qualified radon mitigation contractor. Your state's radon office can provide you with a list of state-certified contractors and those who are proficient in a national radon program.

If the potential is high for radon in an area in which you plan to build a new home, you can have radon-resistant features installed during construction. This is the best and most cost-effective approach in any home, anywhere! If you do this, however, be sure the builder has experience in installing radon-resistant features. The cost for reducing radon levels in existing homes typically ranges from $800 to $2,500. The average cost to install radon-resistant features during new home construction is $350 to $500, but the cost can be as low as $150, depending on the type of home construction. Even if built radon-resistant, every new home should be tested for radon after occupancy.

Carbon Monoxide

Carbon monoxide (CO) is a colorless, odorless, tasteless, and toxic gas created when fossil fuels such as oil, natural gas, wood, propane, or kerosene burn without enough oxygen for full combustion. Motor vehicle exhaust is also a source of this hazardous gas. It is not produced by electric appliances. Any fuel-burning appliance, vehicle, tool, or other device is a potential CO source. When fuel-burning appliances are kept in good working condition, they produce little CO. Malfunctioning, improperly used, or poorly vented appliances can produce fatal CO concentrations in your home.

CO poisoning can occur from inhaling small amounts of CO over a long period of time or from large amounts inhaled in a short time. Unborn babies, infants, and people with anemia or a history of heart

---
DO IT YOURSELF?

**Inspecting and correct-
ing problems with fuel-
burning appliances . . .
Not!**
Only a trained service
technician can do this.
Leave it to professionals.

---

disease are more vulnerable to exposure to CO. Breathing low levels of carbon monoxide can cause these flulike symptoms: mild nausea, mild headaches, fatigue, and shortness of breath. Symptoms at moderate levels include nausea, severe headaches, dizziness, disorientation, confusion, and fainting. Breathing higher levels of carbon monoxide can cause loss of consciousness and death.

While many of the symptoms of CO poisoning resemble other illnesses, such as flu or food-borne illnesses, become highly suspicious if more than one family member experiences similar symptoms, if the symptoms occur only in the house, or if symptoms decrease when you leave the house and reappear when you return. Tell the doctor you suspect CO poisoning. It can be diagnosed by a simple blood test.

Install, Inspect, and Use Appliances According to the Manufacturer's Directions

Prevention is the best defense against carbon monoxide poisoning. If you have experience with such work and plan to install an appliance yourself, be sure to follow the manufacturer's instructions as well as local codes. Most fuel-burning appliances should be installed professionally.

Follow the manufacturer's directions for safe use and operation. (Never use the gas range or oven to heat a room.) Only a trained service technician can detect hidden problems and sources of carbon monoxide and correct them. Have a trained professional annually inspect your gas water heater, gas range and oven, gas dryer, gas or kerosene heaters, fireplace, wood stove, gas swimming pool heater, and your oil or gas furnace (especially before turning on the furnace in the fall). Three activities to NEVER do:

- burn charcoal in homes, tents, vehicles, or garages
- run a car in a garage, even if the garage doors are open
- operate any sort of portable generator indoors, including in homes, garages, basements, carports, crawl spaces, sheds, and other enclosed or partially enclosed areas, even if the doors and windows are open. The ONLY place a generator should be used is OUTSIDE, at least 20 feet away from your house and away from doors, windows, and vents that could allow CO to come indoors.

DO IT YOURSELF!

Never ignore these CO warning signs:
- An unfamiliar smell or burning odor
- A decreasing hot water supply
- A furnace's inability to heat the house or its running constantly
- The appearance of soot, especially on appliances and on the outside of the chimney or flue—indicating that an appliance is not operating properly
- A persistent yellow-tipped flame—indicating that the fuel is not burning efficiently
- Increased condensation on the inside of windows

If you see any of these warning signs that signal a possible CO problem, immediately contact a professional service technician to fully examine the faulty unit.

To avoid electrocution, keep the generator dry and do not use in rain or wet conditions. To protect from moisture, operate it on a dry surface under an open, canopy-like structure. Dry your hands if wet before touching the generator.

Look for Leaks and Repair Them Quickly

Repair any leaks immediately. Make certain the flues and chimneys are connected and in good working order and are not blocked. Examine vents and chimneys regularly for improper connections and visible rust or stains. When using a fireplace, open the flue for adequate ventilation. Keep gas appliances properly vented and never operate an unvented gas-burning appliance in a closed room. Choose properly sized wood stoves that are certified to meet EPA emission standards. Make sure all doors fit tightly. Install and use an exhaust fan over gas stoves, vented to the outdoors.

Install Carbon Monoxide Alarms

A CO alarm is a device that measures how much CO has accumulated, sounding an alarm before the gas reaches toxic levels. Hardware and home improvement stores sell CO alarms, which typically range in price from $20 to $60. Purchase battery-operated CO alarms or plug-in

CO alarms with battery back-up. CO alarms should be certified to the requirements of the most recent UL, IAS, or CSA standard for CO alarms.

Install a CO alarm near every sleeping area, on every level of the home and at least 15 feet from any fuel-burning appliances. Read and carefully follow the manufacturer's recommendation for the alarm's placement, use, and maintenance. For the best protection, intercon-nect all alarms throughout the home. When one sounds, they all sound. Change the batteries on your carbon monoxide alarms once a year, when you change them on your smoke alarms, and test monthly as you do with the smoke alarms. Because carbon monoxide alarms have a limited life, you need to check the expiration date provided on the alarm and in the instruction book. Replace alarms that are older than their recommended useful life. Contact the manufacturer for this infor-mation if necessary. Note: In August, 2009, Underwriters Laboratories (UL), began requiring an end-of-life signal to alert consumers when their carbon monoxide alarm has reached the end of its useful life and should be replaced.

If your CO alarm sounds, immediately move to a fresh air location and call for help. It is important to have the fire department or other resource come out to verify whether the air inside is safe. Most fire de-partments carry CO monitors on their trucks to detect the presence of carbon monoxide. (Because it is colorless and odorless, you won't know if the detector is going off for the right reason. It is important not to ignore false alarms.)

Remember, a CO alarm should never be a substitute for the safe use and maintenance of fuel-burning appliances. Teach your child the dif-ference between the sounds of your CO alarms and your smoke alarms.

Know Other Places Where Carbon Monoxide Poisoning Can Occur

There is a risk of CO exposure anytime you are near a fuel-burning de-vice or there are unusual circumstances. For example, snow can block your car's exhaust pipe, causing exhaust fumes to accumulate inside. (Tip: It isn't a bad idea to have your car's exhaust system inspected pe-riodically—snow or no snow.)

Make sure carbon monoxide poisoning doesn't tag along with you when you go on vacation. Follow the rule you follow at home: Don't use any fossil-fuel-burning appliance (such as a gas stove, charcoal grill, or gas generator) in any enclosed space, including campers and tents.

The same rule applies on the water. CO poisoning can occur on a houseboat or in any other boat cabin that incorporates the boat's engine. I recommend that CO alarms be installed in your recreation vehicles and boats, as well as in your home. It is also a good idea to take a CO alarm with you while staying in hotels as there are no guarantees that hotels will provide them for their guests.

Secondhand Tobacco Smoke

Secondhand smoke is especially harmful to infants and young children. They are particularly vulnerable to the harmful effects because they are developing physically, have higher breathing rates than adults, and have little control over their indoor environments. Secondhand tobacco smoke contains as many as 7,000 chemicals, more than 70 of which are cancer causing agents. Exposure to secondhand smoke is associated with an increased risk of sudden infant death syndrome, bronchitis, and pneumonia in young children. Secondhand smoke exposure causes more severe asthma in children who already have asthma. Other health effects of secondhand smoke in children include respiratory symptoms and slowed lung growth.

For Your Unborn Baby's Sake, Quit Smoking

If you are expecting a baby, quit smoking. Please. The impact of maternal smoking on fetal development is well documented. The harmful effects include premature birth, low birth weight, sudden infant death syndrome, and a higher rate of infant mortality. The longer you smoke during your pregnancy, the greater the risk. Quitting anytime will help, but the sooner the better.

Take steps to protect your family from secondhand smoke. Even if you don't smoke, you and your children may be routinely exposed to secondhand smoke in homes, vehicles, and indoor public places such as restaurants. Try to protect your entire family by taking the following steps.

- Enforce a no-smoking rule in your home and car. That includes guests, babysitters, and workers. Secondhand smoke permeates the entire house and lingers long after the cigarette has been extinguished, so smoking in certain rooms, at certain times, or by a window or fan is not safe. Smokers should always go outside to smoke.

ELECTRONIC CIGARETTES. NOT!

- Electronic cigarettes (e-cigarettes) are battery-operated devices that heat a liquid to produce an aerosol that users inhale. This aerosol typically contains nicotine, flavorings, and other chemicals. The term e-cigarette is often used to refer to a broad class of products also known as electronic nicotine delivery systems (ENDS), which includes electronic cigars (e-cigars), electronic hookahs (e-hookahs), vapor (vape) pens, and similar products.
- The Centers for Disease Control (CDC) caution that although the aerosol of e-cigs generally has fewer harmful substances than cigarette smoke, e-cigarettes and other products containing nicotine are *not* safe to use during pregnancy. Nicotine is a health danger for pregnant women and developing babies and can damage a developing baby's brain and lungs.
- The American Academy of Pediatrics (AAP) believes e-cigarettes and other electronic nicotine delivery systems are a significant danger to the health of children and nonsmokers. In fact, the AAP warns it isn't safe to use e-cigarettes near children. There are cancer-causing chemicals in the exhaled e-cigarette vapor.

Parents Beware: Liquid nicotine is highly concentrated; even a small amount is poisonous. (See Chapter 10, "Common Poisons in the Home.")

- Encourage all family members to quit. Tobacco smoke lingers in hair and on clothing fibers even after smoking, so even if the activity takes place away from the child, the child can still be exposed to secondhand smoke. For assistance, seek advice from a doctor, who can refer you to a local smoking cessation program.
- Be aware that children of parents who smoke are more likely to grow up to be smokers themselves, and parents and other family members who quit smoking are more likely to live longer and be around to see their children, grandchildren, nieces, and nephews grow up.
- Enroll your child only in a child care center or school that is completely smoke-free.
- Frequent only indoor public places that prohibit smoking, especially when your child is with you.
- Ask people not to smoke around you and your children.

Pesticides

Pesticide is a generic name for a whole class of chemicals intended to prevent, control, eliminate, or mitigate any pest. These include insecticide, herbicide, rodenticide, and fungicide. These products are designed to be toxic. It's a no-brainer that a poison designed to kill one organism may harm other organisms, too. Some pesticides can affect humans by causing cancer, central nervous system damage, and respiratory illnesses. Others can have toxic effects on human reproductive, endocrine, and immunological systems. For many pesticides, we don't know what the long-term health effects are.

Because children's brains and their nervous and immune systems are still developing, they may be particularly vulnerable to poison. Depending upon what type of pesticide is involved, ingesting or inhaling even small amounts may result in illness. We, as parents, should be concerned enough to want to reduce or eliminate pesticides. Because there are many effective preventive measures and less-toxic alternatives available, why take risks? Your family will have a healthier place to live because of your precautions. Since prevention is paramount, let's start with that.

Reduce the Need for Pesticides by Eliminating What Pests Need

Like all other creatures, pests need food and water. Eliminate the pests by eliminating what they need.

- Cut off their water supply by reducing humidity in your home (the smallest amount of water is sufficient for a bug) and by repairing leaky faucets. Repair all structural problems. Don't allow water to stand anywhere around the house. When looking for such spots, don't forget water trays under plants or under the refrigerator or air conditioner compressor. (Dripping faucets can waste 2,000 gallons of water each year, and leaky toilets can waste as much as 200 gallons each day! Fixing leaks conserves water and saves on water bills, too.)
- To eliminate pests' food supply, start in the kitchen. No food (including pet food) should be left out; store all food in tightly sealed containers. Clean up promptly after meals and snacks: sweep up crumbs and mop up spills.
- Institute a family rule: No eating or drinking anywhere in the house other than the kitchen and dining room. Don't allow children to snack in their bedrooms.

- As soon as a meal is over, wash the dishes, empty the garbage, and clean the garbage pail that is kept in the kitchen. Garbage that is set outdoors should be put into cans that are always tightly closed, with no food or other attractants around.

Further Discourage Pests by Eliminating Their Hiding Places

Cleanliness is imperative. Vacuum often, and bathe the family pets regularly. Cardboard boxes, paper bags, newspapers, and stacks of magazines—including reading material kept in the bathroom—make good hiding places for bugs. Try to eliminate such clutter as much as possible. Before bringing paper bags or boxes into your home, inspect them for pests. To be safer and more eco-conscious, carry your own canvas bags to the store. Then when you hear the question, "Paper or plastic?" you'll be able to say, "I brought my own."

Plug Their Entries

Don't leave windows or doors—including garage doors—open if they have no screens, and install screens on all drains, as well. Drain plugs should be kept in place when water is not draining into the pipes. Every entryway should be blocked, including cracks in the floor and around pipes. Caulk and seal! Any gap or hole is an invitation to rodents, snakes, and stray animals. A mouse can squeeze through a hole through which a pencil can pass, and a rodent can enlarge a hole by chewing.

Use strong metal grates to cover attic vent openings. Holes should be large enough to allow air to circulate, but no hole should be larger than a quarter-inch.

Destroy Pests' Outdoor Homes

Clean up around the outside of the house by removing all debris—including diseased vegetation and leaves. Any animal droppings in the yard should be cleaned up right away. If stacks of wood or boxes are necessary, keep them in sealed containers, as you do garbage. Create a system that promptly drains rain water from your property, and never leave pails or buckets situated so they can collect water, which can also be a drowning hazard. If pests are a problem, replace mulch with fine gravel. Why? Because mulch is organic matter, which attracts pests and provides them with attractive harborage.

Pesticides and other toxins may be carried into your home on the soles of shoes, where they can settle into your carpet, a place where your child plays or crawls. So make sure family members and guests wipe their feet on the front doormat and leave their shoes at the door.

Use Pesticides as a Last Resort and Take Necessary Precautions

Any pesticide stored in your home puts your child at a greater risk for poisoning. In fact, many of these chemicals are as toxic to us and our children as they are to the bugs. That's why pesticides must be locked away, out of the sight of children. (See Chapter 10, "Common Poisons in the Home," for more information on poisonous products in the home.)

First, read the label, then follow the directions to the letter, including all precautions and restrictions. Buy pesticides that are premixed (to avoid exposure to concentrated products) and use the smallest amount necessary to do the job. If you are pregnant, avoid all contact with pesticides.

Before applying pesticides (indoors or outdoors), remove children, pets, and toys from the area and keep them away until the area is dry or as recommended by the label. The EPA registers every pesticide sold

---

DO IT YOURSELF!

Have a bug-free yard without pesticides.
- Develop healthy soil by testing and then doing what is necessary to achieve the right pH, nutrients, and texture.
- Let your grass grow to 2 ½-3 ½ inches in order to choke out weeds. (Don't let the grass grow too long, for longer grass is attractive to ticks and snakes.)
- Select grass that grows well in your climate and choose plants that don't require much water, fertilizer, or pesticides. Don't buy any plants that are toxic to children or pets.
- Water deeply but not often—about an inch per week unless the climate is extremely hot, in which case an inch every 3 days is about right. Consult your county extension agent for the best lawn care regimen in your area.
- Pull up weeds by the roots.

Where the Ants Are
Flowering plants attract aphids, which in turn attract sweet-feeding ants. To discourage these pests, don't plant flowering plants closer than 6 feet from the outside walls of your house, and don't let any plants or trees touch your house (thus providing a highway into your home).

legally in the United States, but such registration does not guarantee safety.

Go After Pests with Less Toxic Methods

If preventive measures don't work, use less toxic tools to fight them whenever possible.

Ants

You can wash away ants in the house with a soapy dishrag. An effective way to keep ants from coming into your home is to use baiting outside. The problem in doing this is the fact that different kinds of ants prefer different baits, ranging from sugar and fat to protein and carbohydrates. However, since they all seek and need water, water-based baits (containing sodium borate as the active ingredient) may be your best bet. You can also look for boric acid on the labels of bait traps you consider buying. (Please read precautions in the sidebar below.) Sweet liquid baits can be put in special holders that are child-resistant, but remember that child-resistant does not mean childproof. Always place baits out of the reach of children and pets, and follow the manufacturer's instructions.

Fleas

Your pet is usually the culprit who brings fleas into your house. If the pet goes where fleas hang out, it's a foregone conclusion that soon you'll be vacuuming and fussing and fuming over those maddening critters. (See Chapter 7, "Safety with Pets," for tips on keeping your pet clean.) To help keep fleas out of your house, you must first keep them out of your yard. Consider getting some microscopic worms—more politely called beneficial nematodes. These wonderful creatures help control more than 250 pests (including fleas) that begin their life cycle in the soil. Gardening catalogues usually carry them.

For serious flea infestations, consider using food-grade diatomaceous earth. This substance is created by crushing the skeletons of prehistoric algae. (I am not making this up!) When insects walk over the glasslike bits, then breathe them in, the sharp pieces puncture their breathing system. This product can be found in garden centers and pest control departments. Never use the type that contains free silica (which is sold for use in swimming pools); it is harmful to humans and pets.

Before application, thoroughly vacuum the carpet and any furniture frequented by the pet to reduce the flea population. Just prior to vacuuming, put 1 to 2 tablespoons of cornstarch into the vacuum bag. This creates a mini dust storm; the tiny particles of the cornstarch will clog the fleas' breathing holes. During application, follow the label directions on diatomaceous earth carefully.

Hint: You'll have to wear a dust mask and goggles when applying, sweeping, and vacuuming. And you must keep children and pets out of the area until you have vacuumed well. Immediately after vacuuming, remove the bag, place it in a strong plastic garbage bag, and dispose of the bag in a tightly sealed garbage can, preferably outside the house. This is very important because flea eggs can still hatch in the bag. In addition, the diatomaceous earth in the bag can become airborne.

Another treatment for serious flea infestations—and one of the most effective—is steam cleaning. This process kills adult- and larval-fleas and some eggs. However, because the warmth and humidity of the steam may also stimulate the remaining eggs to hatch, some fleas may appear a day or two after the cleaning. Be sure to follow up with regular vacuuming to catch the few remaining fleas that hatch after steam cleaning.

Moths

Hang cedar blocks in your closet to repel moths. Pheromone scent traps will also help you monitor and trap moths. Another way to discourage moths is to avoid putting into the closet any clothes that have not been thoroughly cleaned.

Roaches

Even the cleanest kitchen can be invaded by a cockroach or two. If they have come in with your grocery bags and have not yet set up a colony, you can solve the problem by stepping on them. If the roaches have gotten a foothold, however, reach for the boric acid, which is available in powder form, as well as in bait stations. In whatever form you bring boric acid into your home, it is important to know that it is harmful. While it has a lower toxicity than many other pesticides, neither pets nor people should ingest it. Place or inject the product only in hidden areas, such as wall voids, cracks, and crevices where roaches hide. Apply it only in areas that are inaccessible to children and pets.

DO IT YOURSELF!

Use boric acid powder safely to fight roaches.
- Buy it in the pest control department of any home and garden center or the hardware store.
- Look at the label. If it does not say the product can be used for roach control, don't use it for that purpose. Follow the label directions exactly.
- If you have a pest-control professional, ask him to use a blue-tinted product so it can't be mistaken for food, such as flour or sugar.
- Never leave it exposed on countertops or near food, and apply it only where it will be inaccessible to children and pets.
- When using a broom or vacuum, make sure the boric acid is not kicked back into the air.

Rodents

Instead of putting out poison, use traps for rats and mice, but place traps in areas out of the sight and reach of children and pets.

Use Integrated Pest Management

Integrated pest management, an effective strategy for controlling pests, combines a variety of methods: prevention (such as sanitation and structural repair), mechanical measures (such as traps and pulling up weeds by hand), biological controls (such as beneficial predators), and other measures based on knowledge of the pests. It uses regular monitoring to determine if and when treatments are needed, such as sticky traps to monitor insect activity. Toxic chemicals may be used, but only in extreme cases. Even then, the least toxic effective agent is used. Check with your child's school or child care provider; ask what pest control methods they use. Request that they use integrated pest management.

Chemicals in the Nursery

Have you ever walked into a room that had been freshly painted or newly carpeted and said, "The room smells new"? For someone who has no chemical sensitivities, this can be construed as a good

DO IT YOURSELF!

Investigate before hiring a pest control operator.
- Look for a qualified pest control operator who practices integrated pest management.
- Ask the pest control company/operator for their state license number.
- Contact your state licensing agency (usually the Department of Agriculture) to inquire if the company or operator has any history of violations or complaints by consumers. You will need to supply the company's license number to obtain this information.
- Ask for the service technician's state certification number. Most states require certification.
- Ask for references . . . and check them out.
- Ask to see a current certificate of insurance.
- Inquire about experience. (What type of insect problems has this person previously treated?)
- Ask to see the label of any product being used.
- Be sure to read the product's material safety data sheet; it tells you the active ingredients in the product and gives precautionary warnings. In addition, read fact sheets on the chemicals they propose using, identifying health effects.
- To learn more about IPM and to find a practitioner in your area, go to *www.beyondpesticides.org*, a nonprofit group that promotes safer alternatives to toxic pesticides.
- Request that chemical pesticides be used only as a last choice for controlling pests.
- Beyond Pesticides recommends that you include in your written contract what chemicals you do and do *not* want used. Having this in writing may be the only way to legally seek restitution if the company's agent makes an application that is expensive or impossible to remedy.

thing—something like enjoying a "new car" smell. However, a safe, clean room should have no smell at all. You may be surprised that some of the products commonly found in a nursery—carpeting, fresh paint, new or refinished furniture, and cleaning supplies—can "off-gas" or emit toxic fumes called volatile organic compounds (VOCs). VOCs are a range of chemicals, many of which have hazardous properties. Some are carcinogenic and can irritate our lungs. Formaldehyde is a VOC with a pungent odor. (You may remember this smell from the high school biology lab.) It is a widely used chemical in household products.

A child is more susceptible to the adverse effects of toxins than an adult because a child's lungs are smaller, and children breathe more rapidly. Consequently, they inhale more pollutants per pound of body weight than adults. If that air is contaminated, they will inhale more pollutants. Infants are particularly vulnerable. Because an infant's nervous and immune systems are in the earliest stages of development, he cannot detoxify chemicals efficiently. For that matter, it is extremely important to pay attention to the well-being of pregnant women; fumes inhaled by the mother can pass through the placenta.

Although we are focusing on the nursery, use the same precautions in other rooms in the house that you may consider refurbishing with fresh paint or new carpets, drapes, or furniture. Wherever the baby or the mom-to-be will breathe, off-gassing chemicals can be harmful.

So when is the best time to apply fresh paint or install new carpet or furniture? Ideally it is before you even start a family. I realize this may not be possible, and in such cases, it is necessary to take precautions. A pregnant mom should not paint or be involved with any designing project that will potentially expose her to toxins. She should avoid any recently painted room until the fumes have completely disappeared. If a painting project in the nursery begins or continues after the baby is at home, keep her in your bedroom for a few weeks in a safety-approved crib or bassinet so she won't be inhaling air pollutants.

Keep the freshly painted nursery well ventilated—with windows opened and fans turned on to push the fumes out and bring fresh air in. Do this until you can no longer detect any odor. It's best to perform these projects during the summer months when it is warm enough to keep windows open and fans on. (In hot climates, the best time may be during cooler months, when the air conditioner is not on.)

Remember that if your home was built before 1978, you should test your home for lead paint, especially before remodeling or renovating. (See the section on lead in this chapter, above.)

Air out a room as long as possible, optimally for at least several days to a few weeks. Don't allow your child in the room while it is being painted and wait until the fumes have completely disappeared before letting your baby or child sleep in the room.

Select and Use Paint Carefully

Many paints contain VOCs, which do not stay in the paint. As the paint dries and evaporates, the VOCs are released into the air. To minimize your child's exposure, select water-based latex paints, which generally have fewer VOCs than oil-based paints. Also look for *low-VOC* paints, which are specially formulated to be low in polluting emissions. There are also No-*VOC* or *Zero-VOC* paints. (Be aware that colorants can add VOCs to base paint. Look for low-VOC or No-VOC base paint and colorant.). Even if you use the lower VOC paints, make sure the newly painted room is ventilated well. Children and pregnant women should stay out of the area until the paint is dry and the odor is gone.

Choose Healthier Flooring Options

New carpets emit VOCs from the fabric treatment (fire-resistant products or stain guard), glued backing, and adhesives. Infants and small children are especially vulnerable, since they are closer to the floor and spend much of their time on the floor. Moreover, all carpets—no matter what their age—can trap dust, mold, lead, and tracked-in pesticides. You've probably never thought about the significance of the floor, but when choosing, why not consider flooring such as solid wood or natural linoleum? When installing flooring, the Environmental Work Group recommends to use nail-down or click/interlocking installation instead of glue. If you do use glue, choose low VOC. And choose low-VOC finishes and sealants. You can provide a softer cover to the floor by using natural fiber, washable area rugs with non-slip backing.

If you're planning to use carpet, especially if it has synthetic fibers, ask the sales person to allow your new carpet to ventilate for several days before bringing it to your home. And ask the installer to either tack the carpet down or use low-VOC adhesives. When cleaning the floor or carpet, use mild cleaners instead of detergents containing solvents.

Look for Furniture Made of Solid Wood or Formaldehyde-Free Products

Formaldehyde can be emitted from some new pressed wood products such as plywood, particle board and medium density fiberboard because of the glue or adhesive in the products. Look for furniture made of solid wood or formaldehyde-free pressed wood products. You can also use a non-toxic sealant to reduce formaldehyde emissions. When buying a new product that contains formaldehyde, you can reduce your family's exposure by making sure the product is aired out—with all coverings and packaging removed—before delivery. You can request that prior to delivery, the manufacturer or supplier airs out the product in their warehouse. Or you can do it after delivery for a few weeks before installation. Do this outdoors on a porch or in a well-ventilated, unoccupied area, such as a shed or garage.

Certification Gives You Confidence

One way to be confident you are doing your best to limit chemicals in your home is to look for GREENGUARD certification, which attests to a product's having been screened for more than 10,000 chemicals by an independent, third-party organization. The GREENGUARD label assures you the product has met some of the world's most rigorous and comprehensive standards for low emissions of volatile organic compounds (VOCs) into indoor air. GREENGUARD Certified products include baby cribs, mattresses, countertops, paints and adhesives, and insulation and wood flooring.

Some Baby Care Products Can Harbor Harmful Chemicals

Less is best when it comes to using baby care products. Disregard the marketing hype. Unless special lotions and powders are medically necessary, it is best to avoid them. Aunt Polly loves them because to her, they smell like "baby," but you should avoid using baby powders. If they are inhaled, they can cause breathing problems or lung damage. (The American Academy of Pediatrics notes that published reports indicate that talc or cornstarch in baby powder can injure a baby's lungs.)

When bathing your baby, plain water should suffice. If needed, use a mild, unscented moisturizing soap and choose a no-tears, hypoallergenic baby shampoo.

When cleaning your baby's delicate bottom, avoid wipes that contain alcohol or synthetic ingredients that can irritate his skin. The best way to prevent and treat diaper rash is to keep his bottom clean and dry. Change his wet or soiled diapers promptly and allow him to go without diapers when practical. If a rash does develop, use plain, warm water in a squirt bottle to rinse his diaper area and gently pat dry. Apply a diaper rash cream or ointment, as recommended by your pediatrician.

When washing baby's clothes, there's no need to spend extra money on baby detergents. Just look for a laundry detergent that is free of dyes and fragrances. If fabric softener is needed, use ¼ cup of baking soda in the wash or ¼ cup of vinegar in the rinse cycle instead of chemical softeners.

It is important to choose baby care products prudently. Read labels and select products that are fragrance-free. Always contact your pediatrician if you have any questions or concerns.

Review and Safety Checklist

☑ If your home was built before 1978, have it professionally tested for lead, especially if you plan to remodel or renovate. If lead paint must be removed, hire a certified lead-abatement contractor.

☑ Test the tap water in your home for lead, especially if you have an older home.

☑ Be aware of products in your home that may contain lead, and investigate lead hazards in other places your child frequents.

☑ Seal or replace pressure-treated wood around your home.

☑ Do not allow your child to play in spaces tainted by seepage from pressure-treated wood.

☑ Test for radon in the air with a home test kit. If there is radon in the air, investigate your water by contacting your utility company or, if your water comes from a private well, contact a certified lab to do the test.

☑ Fix your home if your radon level is confirmed to be 4 picoCuries per liter (pCi/L) or higher. Hire a qualified radon mitigation contractor.

☑ Perform regular maintenance and inspection on all fuel-burning appliances and repair any leaks immediately. Unless you are an experienced installer, hire a professional to install fuel-burning appliances.

☑ Never run a car in a garage or use charcoal or a portable generator indoors. Keep all gas appliances properly vented.

☑ Teach your child the difference between the sound of the carbon monoxide detector and that of the smoke alarm.

☑ Don't smoke around children, and don't let anyone else smoke around them. Don't smoke if you are pregnant. Be a role model to your children by not smoking.

☑ Deprive pests of food and water.

☑ Keep all pesticides locked away, out of sight.

☑ Get rid of pests by eliminating their hiding places, plugging their entries, and, when possible, using less toxic methods to destroy them. Use integrated pest management.

☑ If you are pregnant, do not paint or become involved in any project that may expose you to toxins. Complete tasks well ahead of the baby's arrival so he won't be inhaling air pollutants.

☑ Select paint carefully and look for furniture made of solid wood or formaldehyde-free products.

☑ For the nursery floor, consider using solid wood or natural linoleum. Washable area rugs are a healthier choice than carpeting.

☑ Look for GREENGUARD certified products.

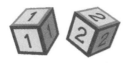

The Home Office

One of the advantages of the home office is that it makes a parent available to the children all day long. One of the disadvantages of the home office is that it makes a parent available to the children all day long. Okay, so it's a mixed blessing, but it is likely that one reason for your having a home office is that it allows you to care for your child. If you must use hazardous materials in your work, safety measures for a home office can be a little tricky. Separating the office from the rest of the house and keeping children out could defeat one of the main reasons for its being there.

An office in which only adults are present is vastly different from a child-friendly office. Naturally if there are hazardous materials that are part of the business or the tasks at hand, children must be kept out, regardless of the parent's desire for availability. For most home offices, however, this is not an issue. Nonetheless, materials that are not intrinsically hazardous can make a home office a minefield of danger to children.

If you are a dedicated do-it-yourselfer, you could probably write some of this chapter yourself, especially after reading the previous chapters. For the sake of brevity, we'll try not to be overly repetitive. Let's consider safety measures having to do with items specifically found in the home office.

Using Care with Furniture and Office Equipment
Prevent Furniture from Tipping Over
Secure all bookcases, file cabinets, and top-heavy furniture to the walls with anti-tip devices such as brackets, braces and wall straps. You're

more likely to have cords snaking across the floor in an office than in other rooms of the house, so take care to secure all loose cords to prevent tripping. This is as important for Mom and Dad as for baby, but in addition to tripping, a child could drag office equipment down on himself. It's amazing the amount of weight a small body—especially a falling one—can move, and you probably have some pretty heavy stuff in your office.

Prevent Poisoning

The same houseplants found elsewhere in the house might be found here, too. Nothing new there. In addition to household cleaners found in other rooms, however, there is an array of other poisonous substances unique to the home office, such as special cleaners, toners, correction fluids, inks (including markers), and rubber cement. The solution is twofold: keep such supplies in a locked cabinet and always put items away in that cabinet after every use.

Prevent Choking, Suffocation, Strangulation, and Entrapment

Talk about land mines! Staples, paper clips, pens, pencils, thumbtacks—even the caps for pens and markers should be kept out of reach of little hands (and mouths). Keep such items in a locked drawer. This may seem to be a lot of trouble—a colossal inconvenience—but remember the reason: that little bundle of energy who keeps disrupting your concentration as you try to work is more precious than a convenient paper clip. (That's why you're at home!)

Keep waste cans in which you toss anything but paper tightly covered, and avoid storage chests. If you must have a chest, use the same guidelines offered in Chapter 1, "Creating a Safe Nursery"; while you're focusing on business, your child may look at the chest and think she's discovered a cozy place to hide or curl up for a nap. Window blind cords are just as dangerous in the office as they are in the rest of the house. Take necessary steps to safeguard your child.

Prevent Electrocution, Burns, and Fires

Here, too, you should protect all open electrical outlets with outlet covers. The temptation to overload electrical circuits and overuse extension cords may be greater in the office than elsewhere.

For the safety of the entire household, resist the temptation. If you need to use an extension cord, be sure to use one that is rated for the amount of watts that will be consumed by the devices you are using. (Add up all the wattage used by each piece of equipment and make sure the total is less than the capacity of the extension cord.)

Consider using surge protectors that have built-in sensors to detect a short or an overload that could start a fire. Also consider an extension cord or wall adapter that provides GFCI (ground fault circuit interrupter) protection similar to what is now standard for outlets in bathrooms and kitchens. Get covers for all the power strips and surge protectors in your office. These plastic covers are like tunnels that encase the power strip. There is an opening at the top for cords of all sizes to come through, and on some cord covers, a latching door enabling you to access the on-off switch without taking off the entire cover. Once in place these covers are a challenge for even adults to open. Just keep in mind that nothing is entirely childproof.

You desire a child-friendly office, so your child will be able to play there. When he's still in a play yard that's no problem, but when he starts crawling, look out! He'll want to play under desks and tables, and you don't want to say no to everything. However, a desk or table that has electric wires under it offers no safe space for a child.

As in the kitchen, hot beverages should be kept away from the edge of a desk or table. Use a spill-resistant mug, just as you would if you carried your coffee to work on a long commute. To maximize the probability that your child stays out of harm's way in your office, designate a safe area in a corner as her play area, or use a play yard. Remember to take frequent breaks so she can leave the play yard or play area and move around under her own steam in a safe environment. These periods will aid her development and, you may discover, enhance your own productivity.

Prevent Bumps, Cuts, and Scrapes

Children are fascinated by things that cut. One piece of equipment in your office that is meant for automatic cutting is the paper shredder. Never leave it on automatic. Unplug it after each use, and store it out of the reach of children. Don't use it when your child is in the room; the whirring of the machine and the disappearance of the paper will draw your child and her fingers like butterflies to flowers. Never allow her to operate this machine, even under direct supervision. The shredder can pull your child's fingers into the mechanism.

You'll want to minimize sharp corners in your office, just as you do in the rest of the house. Corner and edge guards might reduce a busy parent's nasty bruises as well as prevent cuts and scrapes for the child. Sharp implements such as scissors, staplers, and letter openers should be kept in locked drawers and cabinets.

Get Real

All right. You know your child. You know your work habits. As you were reading the above cautions, did you have an increasing sense of impending doom . . . or, at least, a feeling that all this is simply impossible? In that case, maybe it is. If your child, right now, in this stage of her life, cannot be safe in your home office, you must consider hiring a babysitter. (See Chapter 13, "Hiring a Babysitter or Choosing a Child Care Facility.")

As long as the baby is in a play yard, keeping dangerous items away from her is possible. A child who listens and usually obeys can be given her own space in the office with books, paper, crayons, and a small basket of toys on hand. However, it is likely that there will be a period that comes between those two ages when the office is simply too dangerous for her presence. You'll know when that time comes. To know when it passes, do a trial run every so often. Let her become an "employee," with a specific job such as drawing pictures to decorate the walls. Please! Not *on* the walls!

If you have employees other than that charming child busily coloring on the floor—the one trying hard not to color the floor as well—make sure they take the same precautions you take for the safety of your child.

Review and Safety Checklist

- ☑ Prevent injuries by securing all bookcases, file cabinets, and top-heavy furniture to the wall.
- ☑ Keep poisonous office supplies in a locked cabinet and always put items away after use.
- ☑ Unplug the paper shredder after each use and store out of reach of children. Never allow children to operate a paper shredder.
- ☑ Keep small office items such as paper clips, tacks, and pen caps in a locked drawer when not in use. Keep waste cans tightly covered and avoid storage chests with lids.
- ☑ Don't overload circuits, use a surge protector, and keep your child away from electrical wires. Turn off electrical appliances when they are not in use.
- ☑ Minimize sharp corners: use corner- and edge-bumpers.

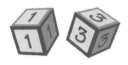

Hiring a Babysitter or Choosing a Child Care Facility

You will never have a more important—or more rewarding— responsibility than caring for your child. When you first hold that tiny hand, your heart will tell you that you want to be with your child every moment. Nonetheless, you cannot do it alone. Regardless of whether you have extended family nearby, child care services and babysitters can be invaluable as you seek to give your child the best possible care. The search for quality care must begin as soon as possible. You can't put off till the last minute the pursuit of a good babysitter, and some child care facilities may have up to an 18-month waiting list.

That's why it is so important that you thoroughly interview, screen, and manage your child's sitter. Trust both your head and your feelings. If your gut says there is something wrong, do not hire this person to watch your child. On the other hand, if your feeling is that this person would be a good caregiver for your child, go a little further in your investigation.

Child care centers range from small independent companies to church-run establishments and large national chains. Some companies, for the convenience of their employees, have early childhood programs in their office complex. Whatever the size and type, the best child care center is one that caters to the needs of both the parents and the children. Don't be fooled by promotion. Ascertain whether a center implements the kind of care it promotes and check to be sure it provides loving and respectful child care.

The way child care centers operate and the facilities they are required to have are governed by state regulations. All states have minimum licensing regulations for child care programs that include health, safety, and sanitation. However, a state license is not a guarantee of high quality. States vary in terms of how stringent the minimum requirements are. You can contact your state's child care licensing agency to find out what rules and regulations it requires. Inquire there to discover if there are any substantiated complaints against the facilities you are investigating.

A facility accredited by the National Association for the Education of Young Children should go to the top of your list, and getting that information has never been easier. The association has an online database (see Appendix E, "Helpful Resources") listing child care centers that measure up to the organization's standards. Be aware, however, that some good early childhood programs may not show up on this list. The accreditation procedure is expensive and time-consuming, and some excellent facilities may not have the time, the staff, or the money to acquire the association's accreditation. In the section on judging a child care facility, you'll learn what to consider as you review facility, staff, and references.

Finding the Right Sitter

If you need a sitter on an occasional basis only—let's say, for a romantic dinner out with your spouse—use a trusted family member or ask a reliable friend who has a young child to consider watching your baby with his or hers for a few hours. You will return the favor at another time during the week. While this is a solution for special occasions, for many families, having a regular babysitter is a must. Finding the right person for the job is one of the most important tasks you have.

Getting Started

Ask Around or Hire an Agency
At first, you may feel more comfortable recruiting caring family, friends, and neighbors whom you know well. That's certainly a good place to start, especially when your child is an infant or toddler. When you must go outside that circle, draw on it by getting recommendations from friends, relatives, neighbors, doctors, clerics, or local organizations such

as the YMCA. If they have no advice or if the pickings seem slim, consider using a reputable babysitter service. The company will prescreen the sitters they send you. Another source is the Internet. There are a number of online services that provide detailed profiles of potential candidates. These services offer background checks, references, and reviews.

If you use a babysitting service, you'll feel comfortable knowing the person sent you for approval has already been interviewed and should have had a thorough background check—from employment references to possible criminal history—and required to complete an extensive application. Don't be so comfortable that you take this for granted. Ask to see the employment application. Inquire about the thoroughness of the background check. Investigate the company first, and then double-check the candidate's references. Better Business Bureau *(www .bbb.org)* will tell you if there have been complaints registered against the company.

Consider Age

A service will usually employ older individuals. If the choice is do-it-yourself all the way, make sure the sitter is at least 13 years old. A good starting age for babysitting is around 15 or 16. Before hiring a teenager, talk to her parents. When it comes down to it, however, you must interview the candidates and make a judgment about the fit between the potential employee and your child.

Conducting the Interview

Evaluate the Candidate's Attributes

The key attributes to look for are maturity, trustworthiness, experience, and responsibility. You can ask general questions to give yourself insight into the potential sitter's personality. What are her goals? Interests? What does she do for fun? The specific answers may not be as important as the way in which they are answered. Certainly, it is better to select someone who already has babysitting experience and a good reputation. If a candidate cites experience, get names and phone numbers and tell her you are going to call past employers. Check references thoroughly.

Know How the Candidate Will Handle Discipline

An important element of your interview is to ask how the candidate handles discipline. No one should hit a child for any reason. Try to ask this question in an open way so that you will get an honest answer.

See How the Candidate Interacts With Your Child

At some time during the interview, it might be helpful to see how the potential sitter interacts with your child. Have some of his favorite books or toys on hand. Watch how the potential sitter approaches these items and engages the child, but keep his personality in mind. If he is very shy and takes a while to open up with strangers, you can't expect the sitter to make an immediate connection. On the other hand, the sitter's response to your child's personality may be informative.

Following Up When a Candidate Seems Promising

Check References

This point has already been made, but it cannot be emphasized enough. Ask for references from past employers, teachers, counselors, relatives, friends, neighbors, and anyone else you or the candidate can think of. When you speak to them, ask if they are aware of any other places the individual has worked—an invaluable source if the applicant has left out any information. Do an Internet search of the applicant's name. Look at the applicant's social media pages if the privacy walls are not restrictive.

Investigate the Candidate's Background

When you think you have found the right person for the job, you may want to consider doing a criminal background check. Let's face it, this person will be performing the most important job in the world—taking care of your baby! Let the candidate know beforehand that you will be performing a criminal background check as part of the evaluation process. Procedures vary from state to state on how to obtain this information. Check with your local law enforcement agency, and they can refer you to the proper authority. There is also a variety of resources on the internet that can perform these services. You should also contact your local Department of Social Services, which maintains reports of child care abuse or neglect in your community. Ask if the candidate has ever had a report of misconduct filed against her and if so, learn the outcome of that report.

Find Out about the Candidate's Health

Learn about the potential sitter's health. Ask if she has had a recent medical exam. If she has not, you can offer to pay for one. With so many communicable diseases—from old ones like tuberculosis to new ones—you cannot be too careful.

Ask about the Candidate's Training

Be certain the sitter is trained in infant/child CPR and first aid. If you like a potential sitter who has not had such training, recommend that she take a babysitter training course at a local hospital or safety organization (such as the Red Cross).

If you must use an inexperienced babysitter, have her begin with gradual responsibilities—watching the baby while you are at home or sitting while you are away for a brief period, half an hour, perhaps. Even if a sitter has had experience, I recommend that you have trial days (with pay) before offering the job on a permanent basis.

If the Candidate Will Be Transporting Your Child, Check the Driving Record

If the sitter will be driving with your baby, it is important to check her driving record. If she has had a DUI or speeding tickets, you do not want her to drive with your child in the car. Ask the sitter to obtain an official copy of her driving record directly from the local Department of Motor Vehicles. The cost is nominal, and you could offer to pay the fee for her. Once the sitter's driving record checks out fine, make sure she knows how to use and correctly install the baby's car seat.

Setting Guidelines

Give the Sitter a Tour of Your Home

As you show the sitter your home, point out and demonstrate how to use all the safety devices you have installed (gates, child-resistant latches, and locks). Show her where you store supplies, such as a flashlight, first aid kit, and fire extinguisher. Identify those areas of your home that are off-limits to your children (and the sitter). Familiarize her with your fire escape plan. Give her this book to read.

Be specific about your expectations and what information is important for the sitter to know. Write these down and discuss them, too. If your child has special medical needs or takes medicine the sitter may need to administer, explain the dosage and point to where you have written down that information. Be sure the sitter understands that she should never give the child any medicine without your permission and instructions. Tell her about specific foods the child eats or shouldn't eat. Also, be careful when explaining the child's bedtime or naptime. If there is a favorite bedtime ritual, your sitter needs to know what it is. What TV shows or videos may your child watch? What books may he read? Does he have a favorite toy? Where is it?

Point Out the Don'ts of Activities with Your Child

Tell the sitter she should never bathe your baby or take him swimming. These activities are high risk and unnecessary. The babysitter should never take your child away from your home while you are gone without your knowledge and consent.

Explain What Is Expected of the Sitter

Make sure your sitter understands the rules governing her conduct before she takes the job: no friends allowed, no cooking, no smoking in the house and no sleeping on the job, even when the baby is napping. Tell your sitter to avoid texting or using the Internet unless it's absolutely necessary. If she's distracted, she's not safely watching the kids. Another important proscription: don't post details of any babysitting job on social media sites, and never post photographs of your child, family or home. Be explicit about phone calls, too. Sometimes her phone will ring; when she believes it's important for her to answer, she should keep the call short. However, stress that she should never hesitate to call or text you for any questions. I always explained that no matter how minor or silly it might appear, I would always welcome the call. Stress that you do not want her to leave your child alone for one second. You expect her to be as vigilant as you are when you are at home.

Devise an Emergency Plan

Arrange for a neighbor to be available if there is a problem. This should be someone who is trusted by the family and who is almost always at home. Be sure the specified person has met the babysitter. Point out the emergency information posted on the refrigerator. (See Appendix F for emergency numbers that should be posted.)

Be Concise with Parting Instructions

Make sure the sitter knows your plans and when you will return.

It won't hurt to have these last-minute instructions written down along with the other guidelines:

- keep the doors and windows locked
- turn outside lights on in the evening
- don't let anyone, even a friend, into the house without permission
- know the emergency plan

Finally, as you go, reiterate, "Don't hesitate to call me."

Checking Up

Be Observant While You Are at Home—Check Up During and After Your Absence

Before you leave, give your sitter a chance to interact with your child. This can be going on while you give last-minute instructions. Observe their interaction. During your absence, especially when the sitter is still new to you, check in to see how things are going. After the sitter has left, ask your child how she feels about the sitter.

How to Judge Child Care Facilities

After investigating the licensing of the centers on your list, you will focus on location. If at all possible, you'll want to be able to drop off and pick up your child at a place that is close to the route between home and work for at least one parent. Next, find out how long each center has been in business. Not only are older establishments more likely to be stable, they are also more likely to provide a broad range of references. Find out how much each center charges for child care. If a facility's fees are beyond the limits of your budget, you will not want to spin your wheels checking it out. Now ask around. What do other parents say about the centers on your list? Listen primarily to parents who agree with you about the importance of safety and any other policies you deem significant.

If you live in an area where the choices are so narrow you'd run out of centers if you used all the above criteria, this is going to be even more of a do-it-yourself project. Whether you have a short list of 10 or 1, there are steps you can take to find the center that is most likely to keep your baby safe.

The first time you visit the center, make an appointment so you can meet with the director. Not only will you be able to determine the philosophy of the center from the person in charge, but you will also avoid taking a staff person away from his job. (This is also a good time to ask about insurance coverage.) After the initial visit, drop by unannounced a couple of times, at different times of the day. Are the rooms well ventilated and filled with light and joy? Would you want to come to a place like this on a regular basis? If you wouldn't like it, your child probably wouldn't either.

Going After Hard Facts

Find Out About Employees and the Ratio of Children to Caregivers
Look for a program that has a low child-teacher ratio. The ratios are important as a way to assess how much individual attention your child will get. The younger your child, the more important this is. In addition to low child-teacher ratios, the overall size of the program is important. Each state sets a minimum requirement according to the age of the child.

Find Out about Hiring Policies

Ask: What is the rate of employee turnover? The answer to this question will tell you if your child will be able to rely on his caregiver's being there for him. It may also indicate possible management problems. What are the requirements for those who are employed to work with the children? A degree in early childhood education and/or child development is preferred.

Have all staff and caregivers submitted to background and criminal checks? What kinds of training and certification are required? Has the staff been trained in infant/child CPR and first aid? You'll want your child care center to be as careful as you are when you choose a babysitter. There should be at least one staff person present at all times who is trained in first-aid for choking and CPR for infants and children.

Your child's health will be affected by the health of his caregivers. Ask: Is the health of employees a matter of concern for the center? Are employees required to have a complete medical checkup? What is the policy when an employee is sick? Do any employees smoke? There should be a rule forbidding smoking on the premises to protect children from second hand smoke. Make sure your children's child care centers and schools are 100% smoke-and tobacco-free.

Ask Questions about Holidays, Schedule Flexibility, and Fines

Ask about holiday schedules as well as regular daily hours. What days is the center closed? Find out ahead of time how flexible the drop-off and pick-up times may be. Learn what happens when a parent is late to pick up a child. Most centers charge extra fees if you are late. Find out if a center can make an arrangement regarding charges, especially if your work schedule does not match the center's usual hours. It is important to work this out ahead of time rather than rushing around with your child to get there, rushing from work to pick up the child, missing the deadline day after day, and always paying fines for lateness.

Looking at Intangibles

Ask about Programs and Policies

Inquire about discipline and ask to see the written policies regarding it. Punishment administered by center staff should never involve grabbing or hitting and should be no more than a brief time-out from play activities.

Health issues are matters of policy, too. One issue you might not consider is whether babies are separated from toddlers. This is important to the health of both age groups. Find out if caregivers are required to wash their hands often, especially after changing or before feeding infants, and before snack time for older children. Are good health practices encouraged? Do caregivers make sure children wash their hands each time they use the bathroom and before snack time?

Learn how the center deals with sick children. The center should be able to provide you, in writing, the procedures followed when a child is ill or injured. There should also be information about when a parent is required to keep a sick child at home. It is important, as well, that the center have a good filing system, a place where emergency contact information on each child is kept, along with a list of your child's allergies and medical needs. Ask what procedure is used to make sure these needs are heeded.

Even infants should be engaged rather than left alone in a crib or play yard. Ask: What kinds of activities are provided, and what is the educational philosophy behind them? How large a role does television play in activities at the center? Are children taken outside each day? What will your child be doing each day? How is the child's progress evaluated? Try to find a center with a philosophy close to yours. It is important for you to figure out exactly what you expect of the facility so you will know what questions to ask in this regard. How the center observes religious holidays may be of concern to you. If so, ask about the policy.

Are strict rules followed regarding who can pick up your child from the facility? There should be a signed form kept on file indicating those individuals who are authorized to pick up each child. A driver's license or photo ID should be checked before the child is released.

Find out if the center has a disaster plan. Ask where caregivers would take the children in the event of an emergency and know what supplies the center provides.

Learn What the Center Expects of Parents

Some early childhood programs require parents to provide occasional—or regular—hands-on assistance with the children. You will want to ask about the other parents who comply with this requirement. Are they supervised? What are their backgrounds? If there is such a requirement, learn the extent of necessary participation and decide whether it is something you wish to do.

Is a parent required to bring food for the child or are snacks and meals furnished? Are the meals and snacks provided by the center age appropriate, varied, and nutritious? How large a supply of diapers should be brought, and should they be brought daily or weekly? Are other supplies furnished?

Are parents encouraged to communicate with the center and with individual caregivers? What are the acceptable ways to do this? Especially with infants and toddlers, there should be daily communication between parent and caregiver. Is there a place where nursing moms may come to breast-feed? May parents visit?

May they drop in unannounced? Never put your child in a child care facility that does not have an open-door policy or requires you to call first.

Observe the Child Care Center

So far you've just asked questions. Now request a tour of the facility at a time when caregivers and children are going about their routine. Keep these questions in mind:

Is it safe? The criteria to help you make this judgment are in every chapter in this book. Look for smoke alarms and fire extinguishers. If you don't see them, ask where they are. Are there dangling cords of any kind? Are there safety covers on electrical outlets? Do windows have safety features? Are there adequate fire exits? Are periodic fire drills conducted at the center? Has the facility been childproofed the way you have childproofed your home?

Is it clean? If it's unsanitary it isn't safe, but this is not a matter of squeaky-clean neatness. On the one hand, there should be orderliness, but if everything is put away and in its place when children are around, it is a sad place for a child to be. On the other hand, you'll want to know if soiled diapers are disposed of in a sealed plastic-lined container out of the reach of children. Is there a separate area for changing diapers, and is the diaper-changing area sanitized after each child has been changed? Is there a separate area for preparing food? Are the kitchen and bathroom surfaces routinely cleaned and disinfected? Ask where the children sleep or rest, and make sure that area is especially clean.

Are toys and equipment age-appropriate and in good condition? Are they cleaned and disinfected routinely? There should be an outside, enclosed play area. Look it over and make sure the facility follows the safety precautions described in Chapter 6, "Safety in the Backyard."

Do the caregivers and children appear happy? Do they seem healthy? Watch how the caregivers interact with children. Do the caregivers get down to eye-level with the child? Are crying babies attended immediately? How do staff members calm a crying child?

Some additional matters to observe or inquire about: Is there a separate crib for each infant? Are safe sleep guidelines followed? Are infants held individually for feeding? How frequently are the children taken to the toilet or diapered? Are first aid kits handy? Ask to see them, and check the contents against the checklist in the following chapter.

Check References

It does no good to ask for references and not check them. Look over the previous five items to help you know what to ask. If a child no longer attends that child care center, ask the parent why.

Following Up after Your Child Is Enrolled

Pay Attention to Your Child

If your child cries every time you bring her to the center, find out why. Once a toddler can talk, ask about the personnel by name, and watch her reaction. Your child's general mood is important. If she is always sad or upset when she is picked up at child care (other than insisting she wants to stay a little longer!), find out why.

After enrolling your child in a program, if you learn that food, rest, or bathroom privileges are withheld as punishment, report the facility to your state's child care licensing agency. And find another center for your child.

Review and Safety Checklist

☑ Choose a sitter based on age and personal attributes such as attitude, apparent maturity, and interaction with your child.

☑ Find out how the sitter views discipline.

☑ Investigate a potential sitter's background, training and driving record (if the sitter will be transporting your child).

☑ Explain the house rules and devise an emergency plan with the sitter

☑ Give clear parting instructions—perhaps written as well as spoken—and stress that the sitter may call or text you with any questions.

☑ Check up on the sitter during and after the engagement.

☑ When making a list of child care centers to review, first check to see which ones are accredited by the National Association for the Education of Young Children, then call your state's child care licensing agency to inquire about the facilities.

☑ If possible, narrow down the list to include mainly facilities close to your home-to-work route. Ask other parents what they know about the centers remaining on your list.

☑ Interview the director. Ask about employees (their backgrounds and training), payment plans, schedules (hours and days), policies, programs, and procedures.

☑ Learn what is expected of you, as a parent, and find out what you will be required to furnish for your child.

☑ Find out how parents may communicate about their child with caregivers and ask about the visitation policy.

☑ Observe the child care center for safety, cleanliness, and demeanor of caregivers and children as they interact.

☑ Check references and ask questions about all issues that concern you; verify what you have observed or been told.

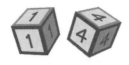

Preparing for Emergencies

You've been through the entire house, yard, and office, getting rid of hazards—locking, bracing, covering, and planning. But emergencies happen. No matter what area of your life you think you have planned to the *nth* degree, events occur that are not expected and not happy. There are steps you can take to be ready. Some are as simple as writing down names and numbers on a form and keeping copies of the completed form handy by your telephones, posted on the refrigerator, and programmed into your cell phone. Others are nearly as simple—a matter of gathering together supplies you hope will never be needed and making plans you hope you'll never have to follow. In like manner, there is something you should know how to do: CPR. All parents and caregivers should take an infant/child CPR and first aid course. It is a good idea for parents to carry the following with them whenever they leave the house: a fully charged cell phone, some form of personal identification, and on their key chain, a flashlight and whistle, which can be used to signal for help.

Although you can make yourself ready, it is extremely important that your child know what to do in case of an emergency when you have become disabled or are not available for some reason. Start teaching your youngest children the simplest information: the first digits of your address, the name of your street, and the color of your house. The ultimate goal is for your toddler to memorize her first and last name, her complete address (including city and state) and your phone number, including area code. Practice with her the concept of what constitutes an emergency and practice till you are sure she knows how to dial 9-1-1 in case you have an emergency that incapacitates you when you are alone with your child.

The responsibility for making sure you have the appropriate supplies on hand rests with you. Below you will find lists of items that belong in your home's first aid kit and disaster supplies kit, which will help you prepare for a wide range of emergencies in your home. All medicines should be kept in child-resistant packaging. Store kits locked out of the sight and reach of children but easily accessible to adults. Remember: When giving medicine to children, always check with the pediatrician first. Use the measuring dispenser that comes packaged with the child's medication.

One of the items in the first aid kit with which you may not be familiar is electrolyte solution. It is given to small children to prevent dehydration from illness, vomiting, and diarrhea.

First Aid Kit

- First aid manual
- Non-latex gloves
- Sterile adhesive bandages in a variety of sizes
- Sterile gauze pads and rolls
- Hypoallergenic adhesive tape
- Cotton-tipped swabs
- Absorbent cotton
- Antiseptic wipes
- Mild soap
- Antiseptic cream (for example, Bacitracin)
- Antiseptic solution (for example, hydrogen peroxide)
- Hydrocortisone cream
- Calamine lotion
- Tweezers
- Saline (saltwater) drops (for stuffy noses)
- Sharp scissors
- Digital rectal thermometer (Do not use mercury thermometers because of the dangers of mercury exposure.)
- Petroleum jelly (to lubricate rectal thermometer)
- Instant cold pack
- Antihistamine (for example, Benadryl)

NOT!

- Don't stock Ipecac syrup. The American Academy of Pediatrics recommends that Ipecac syrup NOT be stocked at home. (See Chapter 10, "Common Poisons in the Home," for more information about poison prevention.)
- Don't buy over the counter (OTC) cough and cold medicines for your child. The American Academy of Pediatrics says they should not be given to infants and children under 4 years of age because of the risk of life-threatening side effects. Several studies show that cold and cough products don't work in children younger than 6 years and, worse, they can have potentially serious side effects.
- Don't give aspirin or any medicine that contains aspirin to your child. Aspirin has been associated with Reye syndrome, a rare but very serious illness that affects the liver and the brain.

- Acetaminophen (for example, Tylenol)
- Ibuprofen (for example, Motrin, Advil) Note: for children older than 6 months
- Electrolyte solution (for example, Pedialyte)

Preparing for Disaster

The need for a disaster supplies kit is not new. People have kept them for centuries in preparation for storms of various kinds and other natural disasters. In wartime, too, having a disaster supplies kit has always been prudent. Today all of us are aware of dangers we might face as we go about our daily lives. Your children are aware, on some level, that we live in a dangerous world. You can use the assembly of a disaster supplies kit as a way of talking about the remoteness of the possibility of disaster and giving assurances that your family is taking steps to ensure safety no matter what happens.

Select a room in your home without a window that will be your safe room. A big closet or interior room would be ideal. A bathroom is a good choice. Choose a room with no outside walls or only one outside wall, if possible.

CodeRED

CodeRED is a free, high-speed emergency notification system that allows public safety personnel to contact residents and businesses by email, text and phone calls. The automated system alerts people to things like evacuations, extreme-weather events, boil-water advisories, chemical spills, missing child alerts, and other emergency situations. Visit your city's or county's website to sign up.

Store the first aid and disaster supplies kit near, or as close as possible, to the exit door (such as in an entry hall closet). This will enable you to grab it and go in case you need to leave and will save time in an emergency. When a disaster happens and you decide to use your safe room, you can take your kits there. Let everyone in the family know where the kits are stored.

During and after an emergency, social media apps like Facebook, Twitter, Snapchat, and Instagram are excellent ways to communicate with family, friends and neighbors. Many neighborhoods have Facebook groups for neighbors only; these pages can be a lifeline during disasters. Word that a tree is down in one neighbor's yard can bring a neighbor with a chainsaw in a matter of minutes, along with other neighbors eager to help. More broadly, the apps allow you to follow key accounts of federal, state, and local agencies that will be responding to and managing the crisis. You'll also have access to local and national media for up-to-date information. (With all these electronic connections, don't forget friends and neighbors who may not be so connected. They may be able to help you, and you may be able to help them.)

If your child is old enough to express personal safety concerns, she is old enough to make suggestions about what to include with the disaster supplies. Food, water, and batteries should be replaced periodically with new items. You might have a disaster drill, with the family gathering in the safe room and staying for an hour, eating some of the stored food and drinking some of the water. Be sure to immediately replace everything that was consumed. This is a good time to check *use by* dates. If food items are close to expiration, why not donate them to local food banks so they can be used right away? Replace them immediately.

Sign up for CodeRED at your city's or county's website (see sidebar.) In addition, consider signing up for the CodeRED app, a free, mobile alert app that taps into the national emergency notification system and sends geographically-based alerts to subscribers nationwide.

An important item worth investing in is a battery-powered NOAA weather radio. (A National Oceanic and Atmospheric Administration radio broadcasts national weather service warnings, forecasts, and other hazard information 24 hours a day.)

Your kit should contain, at a minimum, a 3-day supply. Keep items in easy-to-carry containers like duffle bags, backpacks, or covered trash receptacles. Plan to use only battery-powered or hand-cranked lights, never candles. Glow-in-the-dark sticks work great, too. Kids love them, and they provide a nonflammable, non-spark producing, portable light. However, they are NOT FOR USE by children under age 5 without adult supervision. Begin with the basic list below and add details as a family.

Disaster Supplies Kit

- Baby supplies (for example, formula, jars of baby food, diapers, and moist towelettes)
- Toys and activities for the children
- Supply of essential medications (Check with your physician or pharmacist about how best to store.)
- Books to pass time, great for the entire family
- Flashlights and glow-in-the-dark sticks (not for use by children under 5 years of age without adult supervision)
- Battery-operated portable radio (preferably NOAA weather radio) Buying Tip: Look for flashlights and radios powered by hand cranking so you won't have to worry about depleted batteries when blackouts or emergencies hit.
- Extra batteries of appropriate size
- Duct tape
- Plastic sheeting
- Blankets
- Canned food and can opener
- Bottled water (1 gallon per day per person)
- Paper cups, plates, plastic utensils
- Cash or traveler's checks and change
- Personal identification
- Extra set of car and house keys
- Extra set of clothes
- Important family documents, stored in a fire- and waterproof container
- Plastic garbage bags and ties
- Toilet paper

- Essential items for your pets
- Wrench or pliers, in case you need to turn off utilities

Emergency Plans When Away from Home

You and your family may not be together when an emergency situation occurs. A storm could hit, or your power grid could go out. If your child attends child care, find out if the center has a disaster plan. Ask where caregivers would take the children in the event of an emergency and know what supplies the center provides. Both spouses should be familiar with each other's workplace evacuation plans and what supplies they provide. Decide which one of you would pick up your child if necessary. Establish a meeting place for all the family members.

Go a step further and designate an out-of-town family member or friend who will serve as the call center for your family. If any member cannot contact another, the out-of-town "control" can relay information. If there is an emergency situation over a broad area, you'll have a better chance of communicating with a long-distance call than a local one.

Because someone else may need to make calls for you, list the out-of-town contact at the child care center and at both parents' workplace. For each family member, create an emergency backpack containing the special items that person needs. For example, for an adult, include:

- a three-day supply of prescription medicine
- any necessary food supplements or OTC medication
- a paperback book in his favorite genre
- a small flashlight with extra batteries
- bottled water and nonperishable food.

For a child:

- If the child uses prescription or over the counter medications, make sure her child care or school has a supply to be able to give to her as prescribed. Do not allow children to keep prescription or OTC medications with them in their own personal belongings.
- a comfort toy
- a 1-day supply of baby's needs

If possible, leave the appropriate backpacks where each family member is most likely to be when not at home—at work or at the child care center. (Be sure to keep prescription medications fresh.)

Note: Sometimes insurance companies will not cover the cost of extra medication to have on hand in case of a disaster. Check with your insurance provider for the rules on quantities of prescription meds that may be allowed.

Always keep important information on hand:

- An up-to-date, high quality digital photograph of your child should stay with you. This is the single most important tool for recovering a missing child.
- Other important data to have available: your child's most recent dental and medical records, a current video of the child, a complete description of the child, fingerprints, and a DNA kit.

Review and Safety Checklist

☑ Assemble a first aid and disaster supplies kit. Store kits near the exit door. Kits should be locked out of reach of children but easily accessible to adults. Rotate supplies such as batteries, water, canned goods, and medication.

☑ Designate a safe room in your home and sign up for CodeRED. If she is old enough to understand, allow your child to help assemble the disaster supplies kit and prepare the safe room.

☑ Periodically conduct a disaster drill for the entire family, staying in the safe room for a brief time and practicing any activities that might occur there.

☑ Establish a plan in the event not all family members are together. Decide upon a meeting place and who will pick up the children.

☑ Designate an out-of-town relative or friend to serve as a contact center in case family members are unable to contact each other directly.

☑ Post near every telephone, on the refrigerator, and program into your cell phone a list of emergency numbers and information to give in case of emergency.

Part III

Making Special Occasions Safe

You have made your home and the places your child regularly visits as safe as possible, but you and your child don't keep to the same home routine every day of the year. There are special occasions when regular practices may fall by the wayside. Holidays present special situations and, so, require special consideration. Traveling with your baby, whether during holidays, on family vacations, or perhaps, on a trip to the mall, can be a safety nightmare if you are not prepared.

"Debra's Holiday Safety Guide" (Chapter 15) cautions you about dangers specific to various holidays and tells you how to avoid them. "Traveling with Baby" (Chapter 16) tells you everything you need to know to keep yourself and your baby safe, and to increase the probability that you will arrive at your destination with parent and baby smiling, comfortable, and glad to have made the trip.

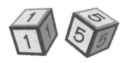

Debra's Holiday Safety Guide

Holidays are supposed to be fun, but often the hole they leave in the family budget takes away some of the joy. Holidays and other special occasions don't have to cost a lot.

After the safety tips, perhaps the most important advice I offer in this chapter is this: You don't need to spend a lot of money to create a memorable event. I fondly remember birthday parties when I was a child. The only expense was for the cake and ice cream, but everyone had fun. I tried to follow that formula for my own children's birthday parties. One year I had a birthday party at a children's library book-reading hour. Another year, we had a field trip to the firehouse. Yet another was held at a playground.

For other holidays when you invite family and friends, ask each guest to bring a special dish. When everyone participates, you'll save money and time (and, perhaps, your sanity), and the occasion will be less stressful and even more fun.

Now, back to safety advice. Let me emphasize that the dos and don'ts discussed in this chapter are meant to help you keep the fun in the holiday, not to make you so fearful that you—and your children—are nervous wrecks. Knowing what can go wrong will help you avoid the dangers, so arm yourself with knowledge, take precautions, and enjoy!

Birthdays

The only exclusively personal holiday is one's birthday. If it happens
to coincide with a more general holiday, such as the Fourth of July,
Halloween, or Christmas, it may take a little additional care on the
part of parents and family to make sure the birthday child does not feel
cheated. However you manage it, you will still want to celebrate the
big day with candles on the cake, decorations, and songs and games.
Birthday candles are the exception to my safety rule that the use of real
candles should be avoided around young children. That's because they
are put out nearly as quickly as they are lit, and neither child nor pet
would ever be left alone with candles on the cake.

If You Have a Party

Before you welcome the party guests to your home, inspect it for potential hazards from the perspective of the youngest person who will
attend. Just as you crawled around to childproof your home before your
baby came, now you can do it with the party in mind. Look under the
sofa, move the chairs, and check all areas carefully for small objects or
other hazards. Look outside, too. Remove all potential tripping hazards
from your sidewalk, steps, porch, and yard. Make sure all exits in your
home will remain clear.

When you decorate, do not use any small objects or sharp or breakable decorations. Because children can suffocate on deflated or broken
pieces of latex balloons, avoid using them. Keep all decorations and
all flammable materials away from fire and heat sources. Be equally as
careful in selecting party favors. Do not allow a child to have any item
that is small enough to present a choking hazard or has a small part
or component that could separate during use. Read age labels to help
select the safest gifts.

When choosing the menu, plan to provide a variety of healthy
snacks. Do not serve round, firm food to young children. Make sure
any juice or cider to be served is pasteurized, and ask other parents beforehand if they or their children are allergic to any foods. If munchies
for adults are to be served (such as peanuts or popcorn), make sure they
are placed out of the sight and reach of young children.

When you buy a gift for your own child or for another birthday
child, keep safety in mind. In the "Christmas, Hanukkah, and Kwanzaa" section below, I discuss some unsafe gifts. Safety with balloons,
candles, and other decorations are also discussed in other sections of this

chapter. Whether you are the host or a guest, keep an eye on discarded gift wrap, plastic bags, and ribbons. Dispose of them quickly, before a child begins to run with a ribbon around his neck. Just remember to keep children a safe distance from lit birthday cake candles. Hair and clothing may ignite when a child leans over to blow out the candles.

The Fourth of July

Our nation, too, celebrates a birthday. The Fourth of July is dear to the heart of every American, and your child will learn to love it when she gets over the trauma of the big, booming noises that hurt her ears. The youngest toddler understands birthdays, and she will appreciate this national holiday more if you explain that this is the Happy Birthday of the United States of America. Those big noises are simply side effects of the beautiful colors one sees in the night sky on this special day.

If we could stick to professional fireworks shows, our children would be much safer. Problems arise when folks decide to set off fireworks of their own. Serious burns can occur when children play with firecrackers and sparklers. Many people consider sparklers to be the ideal "safe" fireworks for the young, but these "pretty little sparkles" burn at temperatures of 2,000°F and can easily ignite clothing. Children cannot understand the danger involved and cannot act appropriately in case of emergency.

Each year thousands of fireworks-related injuries are treated in hospital emergency rooms. Because the private use of fireworks is so dangerous, I strongly recommend that you celebrate July 4th by taking your family to a professional fireworks show.

If You Decide to Use Fireworks of Your Own

In addition to following the fireworks laws in your locale, exercise extreme caution and follow the fire safety procedures noted in Chapter 8, "Fire Safety," along with these important safety tips:

- Before you do anything else, read the product instructions and warnings, and follow those guidelines.
- Fill a bucket with water and have it standing nearby—just in case.
- Before lighting fireworks, carefully check to see that children and spectators are out of range; instruct others to do the same.
- Do not allow your children to play with the fireworks and teach them to leave the area if their friends use them.

- Light fireworks on a smooth, flat surface, away from the house and away from any flammables.
- Never shoot fireworks in metal or glass containers.
- Never try to relight fireworks that have not fully functioned.
- Dispose of burned-out sparklers in a bucket of water as soon as the sparks have finished flying. Be careful, because they remain very hot.

Halloween

Gone are the days when you know your neighbors so intimately you would trust any of them with the life of your child. In these times, you cannot safely send your little ones out the door under the care of a slightly older child. Yet, because we remember fondly past Halloweens with costumes and shouts of "Trick or treat!" we try to give our children a happy holiday at the end of October.

If You Go Trick-or-Treating

I recommend skipping the practice of going door-to-door for treats, but if you or your children have your hearts set on it, there are ways to make trick-or-treating safer. First, dress children in costumes that are light and bright, so that they will be clearly visible to motorists. Second, make sure the costume is safe. How to do this is outlined in the following section, "If You Host a Party." Next, tell your child ahead of time (perhaps while you are making her costume) that you will accompany her right to the door of every house she visits. Then do it. Before you leave your house, put reflective tape on her costume and bag so she can be seen by motorists. (It won't hurt a bit if you stick strips of it on your own clothing. Your young child will love the fact that you are getting into the act. An older child will simply be embarrassed.) Equip your child with a flashlight and reflective accessories, and make sure you stay on well-lit streets.

Use the sidewalk whenever possible, and hold your child's hand when you must cross the street. Make sure your child walks from house to house; no running allowed. Tripping hazards are more abundant in the dark and on unfamiliar lawns. Running increases the risk.

Inspect all the treats your child has collected before he eats anything. Toss out any treat that is not in an original wrapper or was homemade. Also throw away any food that may pose a choking hazard for your child.

If You Host a Party

The best way to let your child have Halloween and be safe, too, is to host a Halloween party. Even at home there are hazards, but you'll be prepared by following some safety guidelines as you assemble decorations and games. The guidelines for planning a safe birthday party apply to any party with young guests, including Halloween. There are, however, some matters that you must address specifically for this October celebration. With your invitations, include a notice that there will be a costume contest and that one aspect considered in choosing winners will be safety. Let them know your own children will be dressed accordingly. Include these tips to help parents choose their children's costumes:

- Masks are great fun, but they can obstruct a child's vision and restrict breathing. I've talked my child into using makeup instead. If you can't convince your child to forego a mask he thinks is perfect, make sure he can breathe and see easily while wearing it.
- I have seen makeup that is both non-toxic and hypoallergenic at [name of a local store]. That's what I'm going to use, even though I have to use it sparingly because of my child's sensitive skin.
- I noticed when I was in [name of store] the other day that they have flame-resistant costumes; they are clearly marked. I've learned that homemade costumes can be flame resistant, too, if they are made of nylon or polyester. I won't be using candles in the jack-o-lanterns, but still, if you can, please avoid costumes made of flimsy materials; outfits with big, baggy sleeves; or apparel with billowing or long, trailing features. The costume should never be loose-fitting and 100% cotton.
- If your child's costume has accessories, please be sure they are soft and flexible. For safety's sake, we've decided not to allow any props that are hard or sharp.
- Another safety precaution I'm taking is to hem my child's costume short enough that he won't trip on it. He'll also be wearing sturdy, well-fitting shoes. If you have trouble persuading your child to dress for safety, remind him that the costume judges will consider safety above all else (including how a mask might restrict vision or breathing).
- I know you're going to drive Halloween-slow that night, but you can get your child in a party mood by letting him be a lookout for

trick-or-treaters who may dart out into the road in their excite-
ment. There will be spooks and goblins out that night!
- If we carve a jack-o-lantern, only adults will be wielding the cutting tools. I plan to let each child decorate the face of a small
jack-o-lantern using non-toxic markers and paints. Your child
will get to take home the jack-o-lantern he decorates. Some jack-
o-lanterns may have cutouts, but you won't need a candle; a flashlight or glow stick will do beautifully.

Christmas, Hanukkah, and Kwanzaa

With whatever customs you celebrate this season of giving, making it
a special time means making it safe, too. Candles play an important
role in most of these celebrations, but my advice as a safety expert is
this: Avoid using real candles around small children. Even when your
children are older, it is never safe to use lit candles on a tree or near
other evergreens, and no candles should ever be left unattended, especially when children of any age are in the room. Candles used properly should be in nonflammable, stable holders, in a place where they
cannot be knocked down. Safer alternatives to real candles are artificial
candles that either plug into an outlet or run on batteries. For battery-
run candles that don't have screws in the back to keep them securely
locked, use duct tape to keep the compartments closed. Even with that
precaution, keep such candles out of reach of young children. When
you leave your home or when you go to bed during the holiday season,
do not leave candles or electric decorations burning, whether they are
lights on the Christmas tree or candles (even electric ones) in the window, in a menorah or Kinara.

Remember, too, that some holiday plants are poisonous. These include mistletoe, holly, Christmas rose, and Jerusalem cherry. Be sure
to keep these plants (and all plants) out of the reach of small children.
(If you suspect a poisonous plant has been ingested, contact the Poison
Help Line at 1-800-222-1222.) Although the poinsettia was blamed for
a death in 1919, recent studies indicate that the plant is not as highly
toxic as was thought at that time. It is unlikely that ingestion of a poinsettia would be fatal, although it may cause some gastric irritation and
burning in the mouth. It can also make your pets sick.

For the most part, Christmas trees are not toxic. However, cedar trees
have caused an itchy skin rash. Pine, spruce, and fir tree are not toxic,

but the needles can cause choking or obstruction when large quantities are eaten.

When purchasing a live tree, check for freshness. The tree should be green, with needles that are hard to pull from branches. Telltale brown tips and falling needles deliver a clear message: "Do not buy!" For better water absorption, cut about 2 inches from the bottom of the trunk and place the tree in water immediately. Be sure to keep the stand filled with water.

If you purchase an artificial tree, look for the label *Fire-Resistant.* Be aware that some artificial Christmas trees may contain lead. Contact the manufacturer to check on your tree. If you choose a metallic tree, use only battery-operated lights. Whatever type of tree you use, place it in a wide, sturdy stand (rated for the size of the tree) away from traffic patterns in your house. Don't let it block doorways and exits, and be sure it is not close to any heat source.

Whatever type of tree you choose, you will want to keep it from being a tipping hazard. To prevent your tree from tipping over, securely anchor it.

Use lights and extension cords that carry the label of an independent testing laboratory such as UL (Underwriters Laboratories). If you reuse extension cords, examine them carefully and replace any frayed or damaged cords. For outdoor decorations, use only those lights labeled for outdoor use. In many cases, lead is a part of the PVC insulation that insulates Christmas light wiring. Only adults should handle the lights; keep them out of the reach of children.

When you have handled the lights, be sure to wash your hands immediately afterward. Avoid decorating with easily shattered lights and ornaments and those with small parts. Be careful with icicles and tinsel, too. If the baby gets hold of either of these items, it's almost a foregone conclusion she'll put them in her mouth. Because they may block the airway or cause choking, as well as possibly contain lead and tin, it's a good idea not to use them on your tree until your child is old enough to know not to put them in her mouth.

The December holidays often bring thoughts of a blazing fire in the fireplace. When children are in the home, extra precautions must be taken—not only during the holidays but throughout the fall and winter seasons. Put a safety gate in the doorway to the room with a fireplace, or install a hearth gate around the area. Never leave your fire unattended. Extinguish the fire fully before leaving the house or going to bed, and allow ashes to cool before removing them. Dispose of ashes in a tightly covered metal container, and place it outdoors, at least 10 feet from the home and any other nearby buildings. Never empty the ash directly into a trash can. Douse and saturate the ashes with water.

Do not burn wrapping paper in the fireplace. A flash fire may result because wrappings can ignite suddenly and burn intensely. CPSC says use care with "fire salts," which produce colored flames when thrown onto wood fires. Fire salts contain heavy metals that can cause intense gastrointestinal irritation and vomiting if swallowed. Keep them away from children.

It's All About the Toys

Of course you want to buy toys that your child will enjoy longer than a day and a half, and you're likely to have a time beyond New Year's in mind. I don't want to put a damper on your enthusiasm, but keep this in mind: Improper use of toys can kill. They can strangle, choke, suffocate, poison, burn, and pierce. Remember the steps we took to make the nursery safe? Use those same guidelines when buying toys for all the children on your shopping list.

It can be tricky to get the rest of your extended family to pay attention to the toy-buying guidelines below, but you'll want to try.

Toys That Can Strangle

For nursery safety we cautioned against strings, ribbons, and cords around the neck, across the crib, or anywhere near where the child is likely to be.

Toys That Can Choke

You've already learned the drill about small batteries, small balls, marbles, crayon pieces, keys, jewelry, paper clips, and buttons. If a gift comes in a plastic bag, make sure it is disposed of quickly—in a receptacle your child cannot get into. Remember: A toy labeled for children 3 years and older should be kept away from children under the age of 3 (or any child who still puts toys in her mouth) for safety's sake. This is not a matter of how smart your child is. Even if a toy has no warning label, inspect it for a possible choking hazard if your child is under 3. Check for small detachable parts and product accessories; security of eyes, nose, and mouth of stuffed toys; well-sewn seams of stuffed animals and cloth dolls. (Stuffing or pellets inside can pose a choking hazard.)

DEBRA'S TOY BUYING SUGGESTIONS

Consider choosing toys made of natural fibers or solid wood. Look for:
* Solid wood toys, either unfinished or finished with non-toxic substances. (Avoid pressed woods. The glues commonly used in these engineered woods can emit toxic fumes such as formaldehyde.)
* Cloth toys and stuffed animals made with organic, untreated fiber fabrics, such as cotton, hemp or wool. Organic fibers are not treated with chemical fertilizers or pesticides.

Toys That Can Suffocate

As your child grows, the list of toys that pose a suffocation risk grows, too. You've learned to remove soft toys from the crib. And you've chosen his toy box to make sure the lid won't slam down on his head or fingers and he cannot suffocate inside. Not allowing him to play with uninflated balloons and pieces of balloons is another step to avoid suffocation. This is an issue not just for small children; in fact, balloon-related deaths are as common among children ages 3 and older as among younger children. If you choose to use balloons, always supervise any play with an inflated balloon. Keep children from blowing up balloons, and immediately discard deflated and broken balloon pieces. Keep balloons away from children under 8 years of age. Choose Mylar balloons (shiny, metallic) over latex.

Toys That Can Poison

While balloons are not usually seen at Christmas or Hanukkah, toys that can poison are in abundance. Batteries can be hazardous if bitten or swallowed. Remember our mantra: Everything *goes in the mouth.* The alkaline contents can leak from the battery and cause a chemical burn to the mouth, lips, and tongue. A coin-sized lithium battery can lodge in the throat of a child. Saliva triggers an electrical current, causing a chemical reaction that can severely burn the esophagus in as little as two hours. The chemicals in the batteries can also cause serious harm to a child if the battery is inserted into the ear or nose. Avoid toys with batteries for small children. Make sure battery compartments are securely locked with screws.

Some art supplies can contain hazardous or toxic substances. When buying art supplies for your children, including crayons and paints, look for this label: ASTM D-4236. It means the product has been re-viewed by a toxicologist. If it is necessary, cautionary information will be included with this label. Do not allow children under age 12 to use art materials containing cautionary information.

Toys That Can Pierce, Burn or Cause Internal Injuries

For children under 10 years old, avoid toys with sharp edges and points, electrical toys, and toys with heating elements. For children of all ages, avoid toys that include propelled objects. These can be turned into weapons. An added word of caution: Don't allow children to handle magnets, batteries or toys with loose or exposed wires.

Swallowed magnets can cause serious internal injuries. High pow-ered magnet sets (like adult desk toys) are dangerous and should not be kept in homes with children. Building and play sets with small magnets should also be kept away from small children.

Appropriate Toys

I suggest you go a step further than asking your family to pay atten-tion to the precautions listed above. Instead, request that they not buy multiple toys. Purchasing one toy of quality design and construction will be better for everyone. If you have relatives and friends who tend to go overboard when buying gifts, suggest that the rest of the amount they would usually spend on toys go into securing your child's financial future. Perhaps they can purchase saving bonds, or maybe contribute to the child's college savings plan.

Another possible gift is one of an experience. It could be a day pass or a membership to a children's museum or zoo, or even the promise of a future special outing or adventure. (It may be up to the parent to make sure Uncle Ned follows through.) Those gifts are for children out of the baby stage, of course. The American Academy of Pediatrics says that when choosing gifts for babies and toddlers, one should consider toys that will build developmental skills—toys that can be manipu-lated, such as shape sorters and stacking blocks. These and baby-safe puzzles are great for developing fine motor, cognitive, and perceptual skills.

Safe Kids WorldWide offers guidelines for age-appropriate toys.

- Infants Under Age 1
  - activity quilts
  - stuffed animals (without button noses or eyes)

- ○ floor activity centers
- ○ soft dolls
- ○ cloth books
- ○ squeaky toys

- Ages 1-3
  - ○ books
  - ○ soft blocks
  - ○ fit-together and push-and-pull toys
  - ○ balls
  - ○ pounding and shaping toys

- Ages 3-5
  - ○ nontoxic art supplies
  - ○ pretend toys (e.g., play money or telephone)
  - ○ teddy bears or dolls
  - ○ outdoor toys such as a tricycle (always used with a helmet)

A gift is not complete unless the proper protective gear is included. Gifts for older children, such as bicycles, skates, skateboards, or scooters, should be accompanied by helmets and other protective gear such as elbow, knee, and wrist pads. Remember when you used to open a lovely gift first, only to find batteries? Everyone laughed, but you knew there was a wonderful gift to follow. Perhaps a beautifully wrapped set of protective pads can act as a herald for a terrific new scooter. Prolong the enjoyment and promote safety at the same time.

Making a holiday safe is the first priority in making—and keeping— it happy. I wish you a happy, joyful holiday with lots of smiles in all the right places!

Review and Safety Checklist

- ☑ Before welcoming party guests, inspect your home for child hazards; do the crawl test.
- ☑ Take great care with open flames—including birthday, Christmas, Hanukkah or Kwanzaa candles; in jack-o-lanterns; with fireworks (even sparklers).
- ☑ When decorating for any occasion, avoid small objects and sharp or breakable items. Keep all decorations and flammable materials away from fire and heat sources.

☑ For refreshments for young children, do not serve round, firm food. Be aware of any guest's food allergies.

☑ Choose games that do not feature small or sharp objects.

☑ Choose gifts for children that are age-appropriate. Inspect all toys for small parts that may come off or out, posing a choking hazard.

☑ Promptly dispose of gift wrap, plastic bags, and ribbons. None of these should be used as toys.

☑ Avoid personal fireworks.

☑ On Halloween, accompany your children to every door if they go trick-or-treating and inspect the loot before allowing them to indulge. Better yet, have a party to provide a safe place for your children and their friends. Do not allow children to use cutting tools. Whatever the planned activity will be, ask others to join you in following the guidelines for safe costumes.

☑ Never leave electric holiday lights burning when you leave your home or when you go to bed.

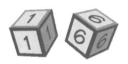

Traveling with Baby

There's nothing quite like a parent's first outing with a baby. The exhilaration and feeling of freedom—away from the house at last!—is combined with the fear of various contingencies ranging from *What if I forget her pacifier?* to *What if we crash?* Between those extremes lie myriad possibilities.

Relax. By planning ahead, you can control most of those factors, including those you have not considered or imagined. Be prepared, stay calm, enjoy the trip!

Traveling by Car

Motor vehicles crashes remain a chief cause of child death and permanent injury in the United States. The proper use of car safety seats is one of the simplest, least expensive, and most effective methods available for protecting the lives of your young children in the event of a motor vehicle crash. In fact, it reduces the risk of death in passenger cars by about 70 percent for infants and about 55 percent for toddlers ages 1 to 4 years.

When should you purchase a car safety seat? Sooner than you may think! You'll need it when you bring your baby home from the hospital, so you'll want to buy one and practice with it before she is born. Vow that day that you will use an appropriate car seat correctly every time you travel, even if you're going only one block to the neighborhood grocery. Most car crashes happen close to home and at city street speeds. Never hold the baby in your arms while riding in the car. That tiny infant, whose perfect little hand holds tightly to your finger, doesn't weigh much, but a crash can pull her out of your arms with a force of as much as 300 pounds.

Purchase a New Car Safety Seat for Your Baby

I highly recommend getting a new safety seat if at all possible. The full history of a secondhand safety seat may be unknown. It may have been damaged in a previous crash; it may have been recalled; it may have been weakened by inappropriate use and storage. It may have missing parts, or there may not be a complete set of the manufacturer's instructions. Moreover, replacement parts and instructions may no longer be available for older safety seats, and the manufacturer may no longer be in business. Even if the seat seems to be in good condition, it may simply be too old. You should not use any safety seat beyond the manufacturer's expiration date; seats are often labeled with expiration dates—anywhere from 6 to 12 years.

The price of new safety seats starts at about $50, but some seats are much higher. Sometimes budgets are so tight that a used safety seat seems to be the only option. If you can obtain a car safety seat only by accepting a used one, please take it only from a person you personally know and trust (such as a family member), who can give you a full history of the seat. Do your research to be sure a) it has never been in a crash, b) it has not been recalled, c) it is not too old, based on the date of manufacture on a computer label pasted to the safety seat, d) a complete set of the manufacturer's instructions is available and on hand so you can both check that all parts are there and use it correctly, and e) the manufacturer is still in business, so you can get replacement parts.

You may not have to take second best, however; there are other avenues you may explore. The Safe Kids coalition in your state or the state highway patrol or local or state health department may have a low-cost safety-seat program for families in need. Every state has a Governor's Highway Safety Representative office which usually knows about programs throughout the state. Since the manufacturers of all safety seats sold in the United States must certify that their products meet minimum safety standards set by the federal government, the best safety seat is going to be the one that fits your child and your car. It must also be one that is easy for you to use properly, so that you will never be tempted to skip a step. For the safety seat to be completely effective, it must be used on every trip.

BIRTH–12 Months
Your child under age 1 should always ride in a rear-facing car seat. There are different types of rear-facing car seats:
- Rear-facing-only safety seats usually have detachable bases.
- Convertible and all-in-one safety seats typically have higher height and weight limits for the rear-facing position, allowing you to keep your child rear facing for a longer period of time.

1–3 YEARS
Keep your child rear-facing as long as possible, at least until age two, which is required by law in some states. It's the best way to keep children safe. A child has outgrown the rear-facing position in a particular seat when he exceeds the safety seat manufacturer's weight limit or his head is within an inch of the top of the plastic seat shell. If that happens before age 2, use a different rear-facing safety seat.

Once your child outgrows a rear-facing safety seat, your over-age-2 child is ready to travel in a forward-facing safety seat with a harness and tether.

4–7 YEARS
Keep your child in a forward-facing car seat with a harness and tether until she reaches the top weight limit allowed by the safety seat manufacturer or the youngster's shoulders are above the highest available harness level.

Once your child outgrows the forward-facing safety seat with a harness, it's time to travel in a booster seat but still in the back seat.

8–12 YEARS
Keep your child in a booster seat until he is big enough to fit in a seat belt properly. You can determine this by easily using the 5-Step Test developed by SafetyBeltSalfe U.S.A. As your child reaches age 12, it is time to make a "contract" to follow some important safety rules, such as buckling up correctly, not distracting the driver, and never riding with impaired, inexperienced, or unsafe drivers. Help them to figure out how to get out of a car when, as a passenger, they see such risks.

KEEP YOUR CHILD IN THE BACK SEAT AT LEAST THROUGH AGE 12.

Properly Match the Seat with Your Child and Your Car

Purchasing the most appropriate safety seat for your child and your car takes thought. Go to a store with a wide variety of car seats. First try adjusting the seat, checking how one changes the strap levels, and then ask the manager if he or she will let you install the store display models that interest you in your car. Most stores are fairly receptive to the idea of bringing one model at a time to your vehicle. You may have to try several before you find one compatible with your car. If you choose a convertible seat (a seat that can be used for infants and toddlers), try it facing both rearward and forward before buying. If you cannot try before you buy, be sure to keep the box and other materials so it can be exchanged.

A newborn should always ride semi-reclined, using the angle indicator on the seat; a 45° angle is a general estimate. This semi-reclined position will keep the baby's air passage open and protect his fragile neck and head. As the child gains head control, make the seat more upright for greater safety (Note: Always refer to the manufacturer's instructions for guidance on how to do this properly.) Do not recline a forward-facing seat unless approved by the manufacturer.

Most rear-facing-only seats with detachable bases have adjustment methods to compensate for the slope of vehicle seats. If not, use a tightly rolled towel or "pool noodle" to fill up the sloped area near the bight or "crack" of the vehicle seat.

From birth to 12 months old, use a rear-facing-only car seat or a convertible car seat in the rear-facing position. However, for better protection, keep children rear facing until they reach the highest weight or height allowed by the car safety seat manufacturer. (This should be to at least age 2, because most rear-facing-only and convertible safety seats today are certified to at least 30 lbs. facing rear. The range goes as high as 50 lbs.) In this position, the safety seat supports the relatively heavy head and vulnerable spine to reduce the risk of head and cervical spinal cord injuries during a crash or sudden stop.

Depending on the model, newborns may fit best in a rear-facing-only seat. In addition, these seats are convenient to use because they are portable. Look for one with an adjustable 5-point harness system. Be aware, however, your baby may outgrow the seat well before age 2 or more. Many babies outgrow rear-facing-only seats because their heads are closer than an inch to the top of the plastic shell, which is the time at which virtually all manufacturers recommend discontinuing use.

DO IT YOURSELF!

Buckle your child correctly in the safety seat.
- Route the harness straps through the correct slots or slide to the correct level, following the manufacturer's instructions (at or below shoulder level rear facing or at or above shoulder level forward facing).
- Tighten the safety seat harness so the straps are snug and lie comfortably flat in a straight line on the child's body. Try to pinch the harness fabric between your fingers. If you can hold onto the tuck, the strap is too loose.
- Position the harness clip at armpit level.
- Do not wrap your child in a blanket, thick coat, or bulky garment before strapping her into a restraint system. Instead, place a blanket on top of the internal harness straps after buckling your child snugly into the safety seat.

When your baby's weight or the level of his head exceeds the limits for the particular seat, be sure he rides in a safety seat that is certified up to 30 pounds or more and continues to ride rear facing as long as the seat will allow. The longer you keep your baby in a rear-facing position, the safer he'll be.

When your child outgrows his rear-facing seat, he should move to and use a forward-facing safety seat with a harness as long as possible. In the past, such seats had harnesses certified only until 40 pounds. Now the majority of such seats are certified to 50, 65, or even 90 pounds.

When the child is too big to ride in a seat with an internal harness, use a belt-positioning booster seat as a transition from the forward-facing car seat to the safety belt. Using a booster rather than a lap-shoulder belt alone reduces injuries by nearly 45%, according to a study undertaken by Children's Hospital of Philadelphia. The lap portion of the belt alone can cause severe abdominal injuries because the bone development of young children is not complete, but a booster seat lifts the child to a height at which the lap and shoulder belts fit properly and safely. Have your child continue using the booster seat until the lap and shoulder belts fit correctly. You can determine this easily using the 5-Step Test developed by SafetyBeltSafe U.S.A:

1. Does the child sit all the way back against the vehicle seat?
2. Do the child's knees bend comfortably at the edge of the vehicle seat?
3. Does the belt cross the shoulder between the neck and arm?
4. Is the lap belt as low as possible, touching the thighs?
5. Can the child stay seated like this for the whole trip?

If you answered no to any of these questions, your child needs a booster seat to make both the shoulder belt and the lap belt fit right on strong bones for the best crash protection. Your child will be more comfortable, too!

Know the Safest Place to Seat Your Child

As long as the child can be correctly restrained in the rear center position, it is generally considered the safest place for a child to sit in a car. Your child can't reach the windows or door latches from the center of the seat and is farther from crash intrusion from all directions. However, the best rear seating position for your child really depends on wherever the seat fits most securely in your car and where you will be able to install it correctly each time. Statistics on fatal crashes indicate that the extent of injuries sustained in a crash is about the same for the right and left rear seats. However, if the center is not available, use the passenger side for safer exit and greater visibility. Regardless of age, every child should be buckled into a restraint system, and all children younger than 13 years should ride in the back seat. Since the most common type of crash is frontal, the rear seat is generally the safest place for children to ride, regardless of air bags. Protection is cut by almost half by moving the child to the front seat.

Rear-facing-only seats can be used correctly only facing the rear, in the back seat of the vehicle. NEVER place any rear-facing car safety seat in the front seat of a car that has an active passenger air bag. A rear-facing car seat located in the front would be very close to the dashboard, where the air bag is housed. The explosive force of an air bag is likely to strike the back of the baby's seat hard enough to cause a serious or fatal injury, usually to the infant's head and brain. Nonetheless, adults should not fear using air bags for their own protection. Air bags have saved thousands of lives. Just make sure you are properly belted and have at least 10 inches between your breastbone and the steering wheel and NEVER put your feet on the dashboard where the passenger air bag is stored.

DO IT YOURSELF!

Do it right. Make it tight.

A common mistake made when installing a safety seat is the failure to get a tight fit. Here's how to do it right:

- Before installing any safety seat, read and carefully follow the safety seat manufacturer's directions, safety belt labels, and your vehicle owner's manual to find out how to lock and tighten your vehicle belt or when and how to use the lower anchors.
- Put one hand into the seat and lean forward while tightening the safety belt or lower anchor straps. Secure and tighten the top tether for every forward-facing safety seat with an internal harness.
- Test by grasping the seat near the safety belt or lower anchor path to ensure that it moves no more than an inch to the sides or front of the vehicle.

Read your car owner's manual to learn if you have lower anchors and tether anchors (LATCH) in your car. In general, vehicles made after 1999 to 2001 have tether anchors; those made after 2002, have lower anchor bars as well. Tether anchors can be retrofitted in vehicles from about 1989 on; if you use an older vehicle, be sure to do this.

Side impact air bags vary greatly from model to model. However, no properly positioned child has been reported as injured by a side air bag. And the air bag "curtains" also help keep everyone inside the vehicle.

Have Your Safety Seat Checked by a Certified Technician

Most trained child passenger safety technicians find more than 9 of 10 seats with at least one error, usually more. To make sure you are doing it right, attend a free Buckle Up Car Seat Checkup sponsored by Safe Kids WorldWide *(www. safekids.org)*, or visit the National Highway Traffic Safety Administration website *(www.nhtsa.gov)*, or SEAT-CHECK *(www.seatcheck.org)*, to find local car seat inspection stations that provide safety checks year-round. A certified technician at one of these events will check your seat for proper function, installation, and recalls. He or she will then teach you how to correct errors or select a different type or model of safety seat, so you can be sure your

NOT!

Never place a rear-facing car seat in the front seat of a vehicle that has an active passenger air bag.

child is protected on every ride. Some of the places where inspection stations may be located are police stations, firehouses, auto dealers, and hospitals. Be sure that anyone inspecting your safety seat is currently certified, *is using the full instructions* and the most current recall list, and has current written material for you to take away as a reference.

Register Your Seat

When you buy a new safety seat, be sure to fill out and send in the registration card for it, so you will be notified automatically in the event of a recall. Manufacturers are required to fix such problems free of charge, usually by sending you a small part. There are websites that can keep you updated on recalls, including the NHTSA auto safety website—*www.safercar.gov*—where you can sign up for e-mail notifications of recalls and you can also register your safety seat. See Appendix D for more information regarding ways to learn about recalls.

Get the Right Extras and Install the Seat Correctly

Merely having the right restraint system is not enough. It must be installed correctly. Carefully read and follow both the manufacturer's instruction booklet that comes with the safety seat and the owner's manual that comes with your vehicle.

Your vehicle owner's manual describes how to lock your safety belt to hold a safety seat. Some vehicle safety belt systems, primarily those manufactured before 1996, require additional equipment such as a locking clip or "lockoff" to hold the safety seat in place for ordinary driving. If your safety seat or detachable base has no built-in "lockoff," a locking clip will either be attached to the safety seat or available from the seat manufacturer.

Most new forward-facing car seats are required to have a top tether strap, an attachment that anchors the top of the seat to a vehicle anchor. All new cars, minivans, and light trucks have been required to have tether anchors since 2001. It is strongly recommended that you have your vehicle retrofitted with this system if you have an older vehicle that does not have a top tether anchor. (Contact your local dealer or your vehicle manufacturer or SafetyBeltSafe U.S.A. *www.carseat.org* to see if a kit specific to your vehicle exists. Some companies will install one anchor or even more for free or at low-cost; SafetyBeltSafe U.S.A. can verify the programs available.)

All new car safety seats and vehicles since September 2002 are required to come with a universal anchoring system called LATCH (lower anchors and tethers for children), which adds lower anchors built into the rear of the vehicle seat to top tether anchors, required since 2001. The LATCH system was developed to help make installation easier and more convenient for parents. LATCH locks a car safety seat into the vehicle without using the safety belts. But in order to use LATCH properly, the vehicle must have LATCH anchors, and the car seat must have LATCH attachments. If you don't have both anchors and attachments, use the vehicle safety belt system. A safety seat properly installed with a safety belt is definitely as safe as one properly installed with LATCH. (Be aware that some vehicles do not have lower anchors in center locations, and most manufacturers do not permit using the inner bars for installing a child seat in the center seating position.) Lower bars have a specific weight-limit, totaling 65 lbs., including child and safety seat. Newer safety seats must have a label with the weight of the child permitted to ride in that safety seat, using lower connectors. Safety belts are designed to hold the weight of a large adult in a crash, so, at any time, you can feel confident that the vehicle safety belt, correctly attached to the safety seat, can bear the weight of child and safety seat.

There are many new safety features in current seats, meant to increase protection by reducing movement in a crash. Look for rigid lower connectors, load legs, side-impact protective designs, features that increase crumple-zone protection, anti-rebound bars, built-in belt tighteners, and extended headrests which keep intrusions away from the child's skull and brain. And don't ignore the safety seat top tether strap, a feature with a long history; it can be a life- and brain-saver, especially in frontal- and side-impact crashes. Furthermore, manufacturers are offering special infant inserts and harness covers tested in their seats. Because seats need to be tested with such added features, don't add items from other manufacturers or make your own.

Today, some vehicles have inflatable safety belts in the rear. They improve crash protection for those using the belts only. However, many child safety seat manufacturers restrict use of the belts with their products. Be sure to check on this before installing a safety seat with such a belt.

Make the Interior of Your Car Safer

First, when getting into the car with your child, enter the car away from the traffic side, and teach your child to do so, too. Check the temperature of the safety seat surface and safety belt buckles before restraining your children in the car. Use a light-colored towel or blanket covering to shade the seat of your parked car. Before closing the door, check to see that no fingers are in the way. Look behind your car before getting into it and putting it into reverse; a small child or animal behind the car cannot be seen in your rearview window or side mirrors. You may wish to consider installing devices such as rear sensors, cameras, or special mirrors to help detect a person, animal, or object behind the vehicle. Rearview cameras are now required in new cars.

Now that everyone in the car is properly restrained—facing forward or backward, depending on age and weight—there are more steps you can take to make the inside of your car safer. Remove loose objects, such as boxes on the dashboard or in the back window area. Even small objects can be sent flying in the event of a sudden stop or swerve, hitting you or your child at the speed of the vehicle. If there is a cigarette lighter in an ashtray in the back of the car, remove the lighter before a tiny hand picks it up.

Use the childproof locks if your vehicle has them. Otherwise, keep the doors of the car locked. This prevents your child from opening the door and falling out, and it prevents an intruder from opening the door when you slow down or stop your car. Locked doors also are less likely to spring open in the event of a crash.

For safety as well as security reasons, keep the car windows closed or opened only a few inches. In addition to this precaution, teach your child not to lean out or put any part of her body out the window. Engage the power window "lock-out" mechanism if your vehicle has this feature. This disables passenger window controls so that back seat passengers can't operate them. Power windows can strangle a child or cut off a finger.

When you leave the car, always lock it, even if you have parked in your own driveway or garage. This will keep a child from getting in and becoming trapped inside, and it will deter an intruder from entering and waiting for you to return. Never leave your children or pets alone in a car, even for a minute. The temperature in the interior of a car rises quickly, going to extreme levels that can kill. Infants' and small children's bodies heat up 3 to 5 times faster than an adult's.

Note: To prevent trunk entrapments, cars after model year 2002 have glow-in-the dark release handles in their trunks to pull to release the trunk lids. If your car is older, I recommend that you get a trunk release installed. It costs about $10. Talk with your child about the dangers of getting trapped inside a trunk.

Be sure all children leave the vehicle when you reach your destination, particularly when loading and unloading. Don't overlook sleeping infants! A major issue, especially for parents of newborns and older children who fall asleep in the car, is the risk of leaving the youngster in the car alone. It has led to the loss of more than 800 young children, especially from heat. Leave your purse, left shoe, cell phone or briefcase—or something that is needed at your next stop—on the floor (or secured in the vehicle seat pocket) in back where your child is sitting so you always check the back. Or you may prefer to place a toy on top of your purse or briefcase in the front as a reminder. Have a plan if your child is late for childcare that you will be called within a few minutes.

Make it a rule that children do not sit in the front seat or play with the steering wheel or the car keys at any time. Children learn from the actions you model. When they have a chance on their own, they will try the front seat themselves and may experiment with the steering wheel, gearshift, and parking brake.

Be a Safe Driver

Don't drive impaired. Obviously, this means never to drink and drive, but it also refers to taking medication that may impair your judgment or reflexes. If you are taking any medication—including one purchased over the counter—check with your physician and read the product label and packaging about its potential effects on your driving ability. Don't take a new medication and drive immediately afterward; find out the effect the medication has on your body. Also, don't drive drowsy. Like drugs or alcohol, sleepiness slows reaction time, decreases awareness, impairs your judgment, and increases your risk of a crash.

Research has shown that nearly 20% of child crash deaths occur in DUI-affected collisions, and more than half of these children, many of whom were not buckled up, were riding WITH the impaired driver. It is up to other adults to plan ways to keep children out of the car with an affected driver as children cannot refuse to get into a car or tell the driver to stop. For ideas, talk with MADD or SafetyBeltSafe U.S.A.

Don't multitask while driving. Driver inattention is a major contributor to highway crashes. If you must talk or text on your cell phone

DO IT YOURSELF!

Be prepared for emergencies in your car.
Supplies to keep inside your car at all times:
- A complete first aid kit
- A hand-cranked or battery-powered flashlight and extra batteries
- A cell phone charger
- A small amount of cash and change
- Nonperishable snacks and bottled water
- The driver's manual
- Duct tape, paper towels, and scissors
- A pen and pad of paper (You may need to post a note on the windshield of a car or jot down information.)
- A car escape tool (which can break side car windows and cut through seat belts)

Supplies to keep in the car trunk:
- A bottle of motor oil and a basic tool kit
- Jumper cables or portable battery booster, flares, reflectors, extra fuses, and a tire pressure gauge
- For cold climate winter driving: warm blankets, a snow brush with an ice scraper, a collapsible shovel, kitty litter or sand, tire chains, and a tow rope

Be ready:
- Have your mechanic do a full trip check of your car before you go. Most garages do this for free if you are a regular customer.
- Have your cell phone preprogrammed with emergency numbers.
- Be aware of your exact location at all times. If you need emergency assistance, you should be able to give information about your location to a dispatcher.
- Check your spare tire periodically to make sure it isn't flat. Carry a tire inflator, a device that can be plugged into your car's cigarette lighter to automatically pump air into your tire.
- Register with a 24-hour automobile emergency service. Keep the card handy in your wallet.
- When planning a travel route, keep up-to-date on weather conditions, road construction, work zones and detours. Let someone know your exact route and anticipated arrival time.

while in the car (even hands-free), pull off the road and stop in a safe place.

Obey traffic laws, drive defensively, and, on every ride, wear your safety belt properly. Never put the shoulder belt behind your back or under your arm or use a separate shoulder belt without fastening the lap belt as well. One day that precious baby of yours will be a teenage driver, out on his own. He has been watching. Teach by example.

Don't Let Your Child Ride Like Cargo

The cargo area of a station wagon or van is dangerous, and the back of a pickup truck is more so. In addition to the obvious hazard of being thrown from the truck—even a child under a truck canopy can be thrown out—there is the danger of carbon monoxide poisoning from exhaust fumes.

Keep Your Child Busy to Keep Yourself Calm

You know the feeling? They're in the back seat, "touching" each other, crying, and whining "Are we almost there?" When they get on your nerves, you aren't able to concentrate on your driving.

Keep them busy, especially if you're on a long trip, but remember the caution against flying missiles. Select CDs, soft toys, books, and games that won't be dangerous if there is a quick stop. It's always a good idea to have an adult sitting in the back to supervise. Remember to take frequent stretch breaks—for them as well as for you.

Traveling by Airplane

Statistically, flying is not as hazardous as driving. You are much more likely to be killed or seriously injured in a car crash than in an airplane. Nevertheless, you may feel less safe in a plane than in a car, partly because you feel less in control. If this is so for you, it is best to take control! There are steps you can take to make the flight safer for yourself and your child.

Fly Nonstop

It is more than inconvenient to have to change planes, running the risk of missing a connecting flight and racing through a busy airport carrying a baby or toddler and all her gear. A nonstop flight is actually safer. Most crashes occur during takeoff, climbing, descending, and landing than during the flight itself.

DO IT YOURSELF!

Wipe out distracted driving.

Don't drive distracted. You cannot drive safely unless the task of driving has your full attention. Any non-driving activity is a potential distraction for you and increases your risk of crashing. Sending or reading a text takes your eyes off the road for 5 seconds. At 55 mph, that's like driving the length of an entire football field with your eyes closed.

• Don't talk on the phone.
• Don't text.
• Don't eat and drink.
• Don't talk to people in the car.
• Don't fiddle with the entertainment or navigation system.

Speak out against distracted driving. In 2015 alone, 3,477 people were killed and 391,000 were injured in motor vehicle crashes involving distracted drivers.

• Be a role model. Your children, even at the earliest ages, are watching you.
• Be an educator. Teach your family members and babysitters—especially if they will be transporting your precious child—not to drive distracted.
• Be a voice in your community.

(Source: NHTSA.gov)

Sometimes changing planes cannot be avoided. Most airlines will provide assistance in transporting your child, safety seat, and luggage. Arrange for this in advance.

Plan Ahead for the Appropriate Safety Seat to Be Used on the Plane

Any child who rides in the car in a safety seat with a full harness is best protected by using it on aircraft. Children who have outgrown their car safety seats (40- 90 pounds, depending on the model) should be secured by the airplane safety belt.

Although the Federal Aviation Administration (FAA) permits children under age 2 to fly in a parent's lap, that agency, along with the

DO IT YOURSELF!

Choose the right car safety seat for the flight.
Look for a label that says, *This restraint is certified for use in motor vehicles and aircraft.* Traditional booster seats and harnesses/vests cannot be used because boosters require shoulder belts and most vests require tether anchors or shoulder-lap belts. In order to fit on an airplane seat, the safety seat cannot be wider than 16 inches. Any safety seat can present some difficulty when you are installing it with airplane safety belts, but if the label and size are right, it can be done! If you have purchased a ticket for your child, and the child restraint system (CRS) doesn't fit in your assigned seat, the airline is responsible for accommodating the CRS in another seat in the same class of service. Also, once the child has a purchased seat, the crew may not tell you to use the seat incorrectly, e.g. forward facing when it should be rear facing. Be sure to carry along the instructions.

Note: The FAA has approved a plane-specific child safety device, the CARES. CARES uses an additional belt and shoulder harness that goes around the seat back and attaches to the passenger lap belt to provide restraint for the upper part of the body. It is designed for children weighing between 22 and 44 pounds and up to 40 inches tall. The device provides a smaller and lighter alternative to using forward-facing child safety seats. CARES is not approved for use in motor vehicles.

American Academy of Pediatrics (AAP) and the National Transportation Safety Board (NTSB) say having your child secured in a child restraint in their own ticketed seat on the airplane is the safest option. Think about it. Imagine trying to hold on to a child in turbulence or in an emergency. Even if you are on a tight budget, don't try to save money by not buying a ticket for your precious child. Cut corners some other way, so that she can have her own seat, belted into an appropriate restraint system.

Inform the Airline that You Will Be Traveling with a Child

Don't keep it a secret. They'll let you on the plane with your baby—and grumpy passengers cannot vote her off!—but they may have special policies for transporting children. Be sure to ask. You may get a break in price, even though the child is, essentially, taking up as much space as an adult. Some airlines offer discounted tickets for children younger than 2 years who will be traveling in a car seat.

If you can, avoid the busiest days and times for flying; this will make it more likely that you will have adequate space. If you select your own seat, be sure to choose adjacent seats for yourself and your child. (You may be on vacation, but it's no fair asking the flight attendant to babysit.)

The safety seat should be installed in a window seat so other passengers are not prevented from getting out into the aisle. (That includes you, Mom and Dad!) And children cannot ride in emergency exit rows. These are additional reasons for informing the airline of the seating needs of your child.

Pack with Comfort, Convenience, and Entertainment in Mind

In your carry-on baggage, include food, diapers, wipes, medicine, and items that will keep your child entertained. Bring books to read to your child, toys, and coloring books.

Before packing, ask about the airline carry-on and checked bag policies. Some airlines now charge more for checked bags, and there are also specific policies regarding what can be carried onboard.

The airline may provide special children's meals, so be sure to ask in advance. Sometimes a flight attendant can provide a deck of cards or a coloring book and crayons. You can accept whatever is offered, but don't count on it. Bring your own!

Become Familiar with the Aircraft

As you board the plane, take your seat and locate the exits closest to you. Count the number of rows to the nearest exits (toward both the front and the back of the plane). In a smoke-filled cabin, you'll be able to feel your way to the exit.

Read the written safety instructions. You've glanced at them dozens of times, of course, but a quick review will prepare you to handle an emergency should it arise. And pay close attention to the flight attendant's preflight emergency briefing. Reviewing what you already know can help you act quickly if there is a need.

Keep Your Belt On

Throughout the flight, stay belted and keep your child in the child-restraint system. Come on! The belt is not that uncomfortable. You wear a belt for hours on a long car trip, and your child stays in her safety seat. Certainly being miles in the air is no time to be lax about using a safety belt. If the plane hits unexpected turbulence and the pilot must negotiate unusual maneuvers, you'll be ready. You won't have to decide whether to secure your own belt first or tend to your child's restraint. You're already prepared and protected.

Remember: Your Oxygen Mask Comes First

If emergency masks come down, grab the one dangling in front of you and put it on first. Only then do you grab the other oxygen mask and put it on your child. Don't even think about doing it the other way around. If your brain is starved of oxygen, you can pass out or get disoriented; in such a situation, you won't be able to help your child leave the plane.

Don't panic! In the unlikely event that there is an emergency situation, you need to remain calm so that you can focus on the directions of the flight attendant and crew. Consider it role modeling for your child. If you aren't calm, fake it. Do your crying later, after you and your child are safe and sound.

Speaking of "safe and sound," you know that rarely does anyone fly from door to door. The appropriate safety restraint system will be needed en route to the airport and, again, en route to your destination. Find out ahead of time if the vehicle in which you'll be riding when you leave the airport will have enough safe seating positions and belts. Uncle Ken means well, but your child will not be safe riding in someone's arms.

Be Aware That Tiny Ears Can Feel Big Pain

What goes up has to come down, and coming down can hurt small ears! However, you can take measures to decrease your child's ear pain during descent. Infants will get relief by nursing, drinking from a bottle, or sucking a pacifier. Toddlers can be given a beverage to drink. The AAP recommends that you consult your pediatrician before flying with a newborn or infant who has chronic heart or lung problems or with upper or lower respiratory symptoms. Consult your pediatrician if you play to fly within 2 weeks of an episode of an ear infection or ear surgery.

Booking Accommodations

Your best sources of information about where to stay when away from home are friends and family who have young children. Their horror stories can save you a lot of trouble, and their good experiences can be to your benefit. You can also peruse travel, hotel, and vacation rental site reviews.

Before you go...

There's one tiny little thing we really don't like to think about ... especially after it's too late: bedbugs. Those bad boys have been on the rise across the country, so I suggest before you book, you check out the bed bug registry, *bedbugregistry.com,* a free, public database with user-submitted reports for venues in the U.S. and Canada. Pay attention to the date of the last report of bedbugs. The hotel may have addressed the issue.

When assessing a property: use your eyes. Looking at the online photographs of hotel rooms or rental properties can tell you a lot if you pay attention. Is it uncluttered and kid-friendly? Those gorgeous upscale resorts with beautiful vases of flowers, bowls of wax fruit and knick-knacks in glass cabinets are not for you if you're traveling with children. You'll want to avoid potential hazards like glass tables and stairs. Wall mounted flat screen TVs (to prevent tip-overs) is a plus.

Ask if the room was recently renovated. New carpeting and a fresh coat of paint might look great and sound like a wonderful deal, but the chemical smell left behind can irritate your children. If you have allergies, those odors won't be good for you, either. Most rooms will have been aired out, but with young children, you may want to pass on that "new room smell."

Does your child have pet allergies? Before you book, check to see if the hotel is pet-friendly. Cat and dog hairs left behind could trigger an allergic reaction in your child. Even though the room seems whistle-clean, pet hairs are stubborn and clingy.

Request a non-smoking room and—if you're traveling with a toddler—one without a balcony. (If you are bringing only an infant who isn't yet mobile, it's fine to get a room with a balcony.)

Ask in advance for a crib for your room, and ask about childproofing material, too. Those curious little minds and fingers are going to be on full alert in a strange place, so find out whether the management provides such items as outlet covers and corner and edge guards. If they do not, you can make your own childproofing kit before you leave home using duct tape, outlet covers, doorknob covers, pipe cleaners, twist ties, rubber bands, and a nightlight.

Check to make sure the accommodations have smoke alarms, carbon monoxide detectors and an automatic fire sprinkler system in each guest room.

After you arrive...

Now that you're in the room, read the fire evacuation plan carefully and find the two closest exits from your room. To help you in case you have to make an emergency evacuation, count the number of doors between your room and the exits.

You've called ahead for a crib, and it's true that hotels, motels, and other places of public accommodation are required to provide only cribs that meet the new federal standards, but it's still a good idea to inspect it carefully, using the guidelines outlined in Chapter 1. If you were told a crib would not be available, you brought along your own portable crib or play yard. For the safety and comfort of your baby, no matter whose crib you use, pack your own crib sheet. The accommodations you booked may not include baby sheets. Large sheets provided by a hotel or your hosts could be a hazard to your baby.

Now is the time to get out that childproofing kit you brought. The tape will come in handy to attach thick washcloths to sharp table corners. Move away things with cords that children can get their hands on. This includes drapery cords, lamps, coffee makers, and unmounted hair dryers. Here's a use for those rubber bands, pipe cleaners or twist-ties; use them to keep such items out of your toddler's reach.

Just as you'd do anywhere else, make sure the floor is clear before letting a small child crawl around. Get on your hands and knees to make sure there's nothing under the bed or other furniture that your child might choke on. No matter how good the cleanup crew, a coin, pill or bottle cap could be lurking in a tight place, and little fingers put whatever they find in the mouth.

Check the bathtub to make sure it has a mat or non-slip strips to prevent falls by anyone in your family, not only your child. If you don't see strips or a mat, call the front desk and request one.

To help avoid exposure to potential germs and bacteria, disinfectant wipes come in handy to wipe down frequently touched surfaces such as TV remotes, door handles and phone.

While it's always a good idea to triple-lock the hallway door, it is especially important when there is a toddler in the room. The door is locked, the nightlights are on. Sleep tight, no bedbugs to bite.

Be Choosy When Choosing a Restaurant

Whether you are eating out for a special celebration or as part of a family vacation, you will want to be choosey when selecting a restaurant to patronize. Ask for recommendations from friends and family and read local reviews. To help find restaurants that are within your budget and have healthy choices, go to *www.healthy diningfinder.com*. The site gives nutrition data about the eateries it lists, and you can search by ZIP code, type of cuisine and price range.

There is also a way for you to learn how safe food-handling and sanitation practices rate at a particular restaurant. Check out the restaurant's most recent health department inspection report and use that score to help guide your choice. In many jurisdictions, the latest inspection report must be posted in the restaurant or kept readily available on the premises. Or you can obtain this information by contacting the local health department. This information also may be available online. Some restaurants have specifically trained their staff in principles of food safety. This is important to know in deciding which restaurant to patronize.

No matter what information you obtain from reports and websites, you can be your own inspector. Checking out the most recent inspection report is only the first step. The box on the next page tells you what the next steps are.

A Bike Outing

Just as you plan ahead for other modes of travel, you'll want to plan ahead for helping your child enjoy bicycle outings. If you love biking, you may be particularly eager to have your child enjoy it with you. Don't be in too big a hurry to share the experience with your child. Babies should never be carried on your bicycle, either in a bicycle seat, a child trailer, or any other carrier until the child is at least age 1. Your baby does not have sufficient neck strength to support the weight of a helmet or to control head movement during a sudden stop or bumpy ride.

A child over age 1 who can sit well when unsupported and whose neck is strong enough to support a lightweight helmet may be carried in a child trailer or a rear-mounted seat. However, it's important to consult your pediatrician first to see if your child is ready. For safety's

---

DO IT YOURSELF!

Be your own restaurant inspector.
Look for:
• Clean general facilities, not only in the restaurant seating area but also in the restroom.
• Clean tables, menu, dishes, cutlery and glassware.
• Servers that have clean hands and fingernails, clean clothes and any long hair tied back. (Artificial nails are a breeding ground for bacteria.)

Inspect:
• When served, examine your child's meal. Send back any meat (especially ground), poultry or fish that does not appear thoroughly cooked. All cooked foods should be served hot and all cold food, cold. When this is not done, it is likely that the food has not been held at the proper temperature.

---

sake, the helmet is an element that must not be omitted. Whether she is riding with you or riding her own conveyance—a tricycle or later, a small bicycle with training wheels— a helmet is a must. Start the child wearing a helmet with her first play vehicle, even if it is no more than a kiddie car that is powered by feet on the ground. Children who begin helmet use early are more likely to keep the habit in later years.

Choose a Helmet That Fits and Is Appropriate for Your Child

The helmet you use should be approved by the Consumer Product Safety Commission (CPSC) and be properly fitted. When worn correctly, a helmet can reduce the risk of head injury by 85 percent. A lightweight toddler helmet should always be worn by a young passenger to prevent or minimize head injury. It is, of necessity, lightweight, because a toddler's neck is not strong enough for a regular helmet. The correct toddler's helmet will come down low around the back of the head for more coverage. All bicycle helmets sold today must meet the CPSC standard. Look for a sticker inside the helmet. If the smallest toddler's helmet you can find is too big for your child, even if he is older than a year, wait until he grows big enough to fit into it.

DO IT YOURSELF!

Correct helmet fit is essential.
- Use foam pads inside the helmet so that it fits snugly, like a cap, and does not move on the head.
- Fit the helmet so the front is just above the top of the eyebrows.
- Adjust the two side straps so they meet in a *V* right under each ear. The adjustment buckle should be just below the ear lobe.
- Adjust the chin strap snugly under the chin. Make it tight enough so the helmet pulls down when the child opens his mouth. Being able to fit one finger between the strap and the chin is a good guide.
- Teach your child to wear the helmet correctly.
- Check often to make sure straps stay snug and the helmet stays level on the head.

The sidebar tells you how to fit your child's helmet. Don't forget that your helmet should fit correctly, too. The helmet should sit level on your head and be no more than two fingers above your eyebrows and fit snug like a cap. If need be, use the adjusting pads that came with the helmet or the adjusting band for the proper fit. Look at your ears; the side straps should be in front and behind the ears, and the buckle should be just below the ear lobe. Open your mouth as wide as possible; if you can't feel the helmet hug your head, tighten those straps. You shouldn't be able to fit more than a finger's width between the strap and the chin— that's the wearer's finger, not yours. Teach your child to do this exercise with you; have fun while learning.

If you let your child pick out the helmet, he will be more likely to wear it. Another way to maximize his helmet use is for him to see you always wearing yours. In addition to role modeling, you must keep yourself safe, so you can be there to care for your child.

Don't Reuse a Damaged Helmet

Bicycle helmets are designed for one fall. Any helmet that has been through a crash should be replaced, because foam crush and even invisible cracks can greatly reduce its effectiveness in preventing injuries. Some manufacturers will replace helmets free of charge, so contact the manufacturer if your helmet has been involved in a crash.

Choose ASTM-Approved Seating for Bicycling with Your Child

If you decide to purchase a carrier for the bike, I highly recommend that you have the seat installed at a bike store. Whether you purchase a trailer or a bike-mounted child seat, check to be sure it has a sticker saying it meets ASTM safety standards. Be sure the trailer or carrier has a rear reflector. Also look at the weight rating. Usually a bike-mounted seat can safely hold only 40 pounds or less. On the other hand, some trailers are designed to carry more than one child or loads up to 100 pounds.

Whichever choice you make, remember to purchase equipment from a reputable bicycle shop and to carefully read the instruction manual. Here are features your rear-mounted child seat should have:

- a high back
- a sturdy shoulder harness and lap belt that will fit snugly
- spoke guards that will prevent feet and hands from being caught in the wheels

A rear-mounted seat brings your child closer to you when cycling, but when you ride this way your bicycle's center of gravity shifts, making the bike less stable. After you have attached a child seat to your bicycle, making sure it is securely attached over the rear wheel, practice without your child. Get something like a bag of potatoes that approximates your child's weight and strap it in. Get used to the change in the way you balance as you ride. Only a skilled rider should carry a child on a bike. Keep in mind that if your child falls asleep in the seat, her weight is likely to shift, especially on turns. This will affect your steering.

Practice getting on and off the bike without swinging your leg over the child seat. This skill is very important if you have to dismount in an emergency situation. Never leave your bicycle unattended with your child in the child seat. If the bicycle falls over (which is likely if you aren't on it), your child will fall about 4 feet to the pavement.

A trailer offers a more stable and secure environment for your toddler. The extra space can also be valuable for bringing toys, drinks, snacks, extra clothing, and other supplies. When shopping for a bike trailer, be sure the trailer has a shoulder harness and lap belt to secure your child, mesh windows, and a swivel hinge to prevent the trailer from tipping over if the bicycle falls. In addition, the trailer should be designed with a roll bar that will protect your child in the unlikely event the trailer tips over. When pulling a trailer, be cognizant of the trailer's width, from wheel to wheel. This is of particular importance if you are riding on a sidewalk and have to go around an obstacle, such as a light pole, or if there is a drop-off at the edge of the sidewalk or path. You don't want the trailer to go off the edge and tip into traffic. Because trailers are low to the ground, they are difficult for motorists to see, so a 6-foot orange or red flag for greater visibility is a must. This is especially important for motorists who want to cross your path; without the flag they won't be expecting the additional length and may turn too soon behind you.

Regardless of whether you use a bicycle-mounted seat or pull a trailer, it is important to remember that you have extra weight on the bike, and it will take longer to stop and start. If you have gears on your bike and you don't know how to use them, this is the time to learn. Make sure the brakes on your bike are in good working order. Practice turns first without the child in tow. Turns have to be slower and wider. Always try to ride with another adult behind the trailer.

Avoid riding at dawn, dusk, or night. Be sure you and your child wear appropriate footwear, and do not wear clothes that can get caught in rotating parts. Wear bright, fluorescent clothing that makes you more visible in daylight, and attach reflective materials on the bike and trailer. Ride only in safe areas like parks, bike paths and in quiet neighborhoods where there is little risk of encountering moving vehicles. Select smooth paths, avoid bumpy rides.

Be extra careful near driveways and intersections; watch for right- and left-turning motorists. Avoid busy thoroughfares and bad weather, and ride with maximum caution and at a reduced speed. Obey all traffic laws. If the child screams a lot or is too fidgety, give up cycling with him for a while. Try again when he is older.

Once your toddler is old enough to understand, let her know from time to time as you ride what safety measures you are taking. You will want to do this anytime you are out together, whether you are on the bicycle or walking or grocery shopping. Always keep in mind that your child will one day be doing this alone. Let her know how to look for cars, whether parked or moving, and show her how to modify her speed when others are walking or biking nearby. All this is a teaching-learning period. A toddler is not knowledgeable or wise enough to ride or walk

NOT!

Togetherness on exercise equipment . . .?
You may enjoy bike outings with your child so much you're tempted to
have her join you on your exercise equipment, especially on a rainy day
when you can't go outside. Don't do it!
    Exercise equipment has weights that can fall and mechanisms that move
and pinch. And she can fall off. (There is no safety seat on your equipment
that should tell you something.) When the equipment is not in use, lock
it away from exploring hands and feet.

alone away from home, but learning can take place long before that
time comes.
    After the ride is over, be sure the helmet is removed before your child
goes off to play, especially on playground equipment. The helmet strap
poses a strangulation hazard.

Not for Fun: The Shopping Cart

Shopping carts in the grocery store are for carrying items you wish to
purchase. Coincidentally, the cart offers a place for your child to sit.
You don't want a toddler underfoot at the grocery store, but the shopping cart is not a babysitter, and it is not a toy. There are certain rules
of safety with this vehicle, just as there are with others.

The Best Choice: Leave Baby at Home

If possible, leave children at home with another adult. Don't make a
trip to the grocery store an outing if you have a choice. If you must
bring children along, the next best thing is to bring an adult with you
to help watch the children. It's a tall order to keep a hand and an eye on
the cart while taking items off the shelves and looking at your shopping
list. Consider making the trip to the store a family affair if you have a
spouse who is able to go with you. In lieu of a cooperative spouse, perhaps a friend can accompany you. A second set of eyes and hands will
make shopping and watching a lot easier.
    Another option, if you don't have a lot to buy, is to put your child
in a stroller or wagon with a basket for items you will purchase. If your
child is older (well out of the toddler stage), praise her extravagantly for

walking close to you—not pulling things off the shelves and not trying to hang off the cart. (Note: this can be a lot of work!)

If you must face the shopping cart alone with your child, here are some tips to keep him safe.

Choose a Cart That Is Not Defective

The cart has a narrow wheel base in relation to its height, so the center of gravity is affected when you put a child in it. For this reason you do not want to set your child's infant seat on top of it. The center of gravity would be affected even more, thus increasing the chances of tipping. Before you put your child in the seat, make sure the cart is not defective. You have probably, at some time, quickly chosen a cart and then, halfway down the aisle, discovered a rickety wheel. It's annoying to go *clackety-clack* all over the store, but annoying is not the word for it if your child is in the cart. If the cart is wobbly or unstable in any way, find another cart before putting your child at risk.

Wipe the Cart

Some stores provide sanitizing wipes, but if the store where you shop does not do this, bring your own sanitizer to wipe down the cart handle and cart seat before seating your baby. This is important because sometimes parents have little choice but to bring a sick child with them to shop, and the handles and seat of the cart are prone to high germ exposure. As soon as you get home, wash your hands and your child's hands.

Strap Your Baby into the Seat Section of the Cart and Stay on Duty

If the store where you shop does not have safety belts, buy your own and bring it every time you shop with your child. At the store, buckle your child in snugly and make sure her legs are placed through the leg openings. Even after taking that precaution, do not leave her in the cart alone. Stay right with it; don't walk away from it—not for a second. Don't allow another child to push it; don't allow an older child to hang onto the cart at the front or sides; and don't allow your child to stand up in the cart. Falls from shopping carts are one of the leading causes of head injuries to young children. Keep children away from the wheels where little fingers can get pinched. Most injuries happen when a child has stood up in a cart or was climbing on it; a fall in the store means a hard landing. If the child is old enough, have him walk beside you, and no hanging onto the cart!

Some stores offer carts with safer designs and a lower center of gravity. One example is the cart with a small model car in front of the cart. Here, too, you will want to use that sanitizer.

Review and Safety Checklist

☑ Before you purchase a car safety seat, match it with your car and by your child's size and age; make sure it is installed properly.

☑ Never place a rear-facing child safety seat in the front seat of a car that has an active passenger air bag. And never put any child in a cargo area.

☑ Remove potential flying missiles from inside the car.

☑ Be a safe driver and a good role model: don't drive while impaired and always wear your safety belt.

☑ Fly on a nonstop flight if possible.

☑ Let the airline know ahead of time that your child is flying with you.

☑ Any child who rides in the car in a safety seat with a full harness is best protected by using it on an aircraft.

☑ Pack a carry-on for comfort, convenience, and entertainment on the plane.

☑ When onboard, become familiar with the aircraft, keep your belt on, and if oxygen is needed, put your mask on first.

☑ Never carry a child under the age of 1 on your bicycle, whether in a bicycle seat, a child trailer, or any other carrier.

☑ Consult your pediatrician before taking your child biking to see if the child is ready.

☑ For bicycling with your child, choose helmets that fit—one for you and one for your child. Both you and your child should always wear helmets while biking.

☑ Choose safe and appropriate bicycle seating for your child, either a child trailer or a rear-mounted seat.

☑ Ride only in safe areas, select smooth paths and ride at a reduced speed.

☑ In stores, find a stable cart and buckle your baby into it. Don't use an infant seat on top of the cart's seat.

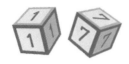

Final Thoughts

Go Back to Basics for Healthy Living!

In today's fast-paced world, the environment can affect your children more than you do. It's easy to feel you have no control. Parents may find themselves trying to take control by driving their children to one activity after another, always rushing, never taking time just to "hang out," as the kids say. The answer, however, does not lie in that kind of frenzied activity. There are ways to exert your influence over your children while enjoying being with them in a more relaxed atmosphere. In fact, in today's economy, families are looking for ways to fill in the gaps left by having to give up expensive activities. There are plenty of ways to have fun without spending a lot of money. Here are simple tactics to help you ground your children in your values and promote healthy living for the entire family.

Everyone has to eat, so use that fact to get the family together once a day. If that is impossible for your family, try to do it at least once a week. Turn off the TV, cell phone, computer, and other electronic devices and sit at the table. Yes, I said cell phone, and that means you. As parents we are role models, and removing our cell phone and other distractions will teach our young children to be more present in the moment. When they are older and have their own phones and electronic devices, they will take it for granted that such distractions are not to be used at the table. Encourage—but don't require—each child to tell something funny, sad, scary, boring or aggravating, and be sure you have a story, too. Allow each person at the table to comment, but no negative judgments allowed!

An essential part of your child's development is play; it helps children learn and grow physically, mentally, socially and emotionally. You'll start

SUPERVISE CHILDREN'S MEDIA USE*

- Develop a family media plan that takes into account the health, education and entertainment needs of each child as well as needs of the entire family.
- For children younger than 18 months, avoid use of screen media other than video-chatting. Parents of children 18 to 24 months of age who want to introduce digital media should choose high-quality programming and watch it with their children to help them understand what they're seeing.
- For children ages 2 to 5 years, limit screen use to one hour per day of high-quality programs. Parents should co-view media with children to help them understand what they are seeing and apply it to the world around them.
- For children ages 6 and older, place consistent limits on the time spent using media and on types of media used; make sure media devices do not take the place of adequate sleep, physical activity and other behaviors essential to good health.
- Designate media-free times together, such as dinner or driving, as well as media-free locations at home, such as bedrooms.
- Have ongoing communication about online citizenship and safety, including treating others with respect online and offline.
- Use the Family Media Use Plan tool, launched on *www .HealthyChildren.org.*

*Recommendations 2 through 6 from the American Academy of Pediatrics, 10/21/2016, *www.aap.org/en-us/about-the-aap/aap-press-room /pages/american-academy-of-pediatrics-announces-new-recommendations-for -childrens-media-use.aspx*

early, with simple and fun games that require only you and your child; no tools needed—clapping games, such as Pat-A-Cake, and songs that combine hand gestures and music, are fun for toddlers. Peek-A-Boo, of course, is the basic game for the youngest child, and it will continue to delight her into her toddler years.

Reading is another kind of play, and research shows it's never too early to start enjoying books with your baby. Books are an integral part of your child's language development, so it's wise to introduce the routine of a bedtime story as early as possible. Be interactive as you read; your child will have more fun and learn more.

Read to your child every day as long as he cannot read for himself. When he is a beginning reader, let him read to you. You can attend reading hours at the library or borrow books to take home. The library is also a good source of music to which you can sing along with your child. Let singing be a way of life. It's a way to share good feelings.

Create family rituals and traditions. In addition to any religious practices you may wish to conduct at home, you can set aside certain nights for family activities. Have a joke night once a week; it will take only a few minutes, but going to bed smiling does wonders for the disposition. When your children are older, you can borrow funny movies from the library. Laughter will bring your family together as nothing else can.

Take frequent walks as a family, going to parks and nature trails or just around the block. Walking together builds camaraderie, and you'll be surprised at some of the comments your children will make. It's a great way to get to know your children. They will also enjoy creating special foods with you alone and as a family, and the time you spend together making holiday decorations will stay with them forever.

Teach your child to help others by volunteering and donating (school drives, holiday food banks). This is another way to instill your values into your child.

Let your children know the significance of family and each child's importance in your life. Decorate your home with family photographs and children's artwork. Play together with a toy, craft or game, and give some one-on-one time with each child doing what that child enjoys most.

I leave you with one of my favorite quotes:

> *A hundred years from now*
> *It will not matter*
> *What my bank account was,*
> *The sort of house I lived in,*
> *Or the kind of car I drove.*
> *But the world may be different,*
> *because I was important in the life of a child.*
>
> (excerpt from
> *"Within My Power"* by Forest Witcraft)

✦

Appendices

A Room-by-Room Checklist

As was mentioned in the introduction to Part II, "Safety Measures for Every Living Space," you must learn to look at your home from your child's perspective, getting down on your hands and knees, crawling around each room. However, there is more to this concept: You must also consider whatever the child's perspective will be at the next stage. As soon as your child enters a new stage of development, begin preparing for the next, even when it means going out and buying new items. For example, you should have gates ready for installation before your child becomes mobile.

Once you get into the do-it-yourself mode, you'll begin to notice safety hazards outside your home. Anywhere you take your child—the homes of friends and relatives or child care center—you'll want to carefully scan for anything that might cause harm. I don't recommend walking into someone's home and scooping up items as though you were a robotic hazard-crane, but there are polite ways to ask that certain dangerous items be removed. Certainly at your child care center, the personnel should be glad for your input.

Any recalled equipment your child may use is a potential danger, and you should not be shy about looking for such items at the child care center, as well as at home. Inform your child care providers, family, and friends that they can obtain recall information on the government website *www.recalls.gov*, mentioned in Chapter 5. See Appendix D, "Recall Information," for ways to contact specific government agencies.

Do-It-Yourself Safety Throughout the House
Install It!

☑ Install smoke alarms in every bedroom, outside each separate sleeping area, and on every level of the home, including the basement. Change batteries once every year; test them monthly; replace the units every 10 years.

☑ Install a multipurpose fire extinguisher in the kitchen, where most fires occur. It's also a good idea to put a fire extinguisher in the basement and workshop. Learn how to use it before an emergency occurs.

☑ Install a carbon monoxide alarm in every sleeping area, on every level of the home and at least 15 feet from any fuel-burning appliance.

☑ Install ground fault circuit interrupters (GFCIs) if you do not already have them.

☑ Place safety covers over all electrical outlets.

☑ Anchor top-heavy furniture to the wall with anti-tip devices such as brackets, braces, and wall straps.

☑ Secure your TVs. Televisions that are not wall mounted should be anchored to the wall and stand.

☑ Install window safety devices on every window in your home, especially windows on the second story and above. Use quick-release mechanisms on any windows that are part of your fire-escape plans. Check local building and fire codes first.

☑ Install only cordless window coverings in your home.

Lock It!

☑ Keep matches and cigarette lighters out of children's sight and reach.

☑ Keep tobacco and e-cigarette products, especially liquid nicotine out of children's sight and reach.

☑ Keep button batteries (such as found in key fobs and remote controls) out of children's sight and reach.

☑ Keep children away from exercise equipment; store and lock it away after each use.

Test It!

☑ Make sure all fuel-burning appliances are properly vented and inspected annually.

☑ Test your home for lead-based paint if it was built before 1978. Ask your pediatrician or health department if your child should be tested for lead.

☑ Test your home for radon. (Call 800-557-2366 for more information.)

☑ Check your home to make sure no recalled products are being used.

Do It!

☑ Plan escape routes and conduct fire drills with the entire family.

☑ Dress children in flame-resistant or snug-fitting sleepwear.

☑ Enforce a no-smoking rule in your home and car.

☑ Eliminate sources of mold, dust, and insects such as cockroaches to help prevent asthma attacks. Keep pets and their bedding clean and off the furniture if possible.

☑ Use door stops and door holders to keep little fingers from being pinched.

☑ Post emergency telephone numbers—including the Poison Help line number (1-800-222-1222)—near every phone in the house and on the refrigerator.

☑ Enroll in an infant/child CPR and first aid course; every parent and caregiver should do so.

Not!

☑ Never leave your young child in or around water without close and constant supervision. These include bathtubs, toilets, liquid-filled buckets, coolers with melting ice, diaper pails, wading pools, swimming pools, hot tubs, fountains, wells, canals, ponds, lakes, or other bodies of water.

Do-It-Yourself Safety in the Kitchen

Install It!

☑ Install guards on stove knobs.

Lock It!

☑ Store household cleaning products, pet supplies, medicine, supplements, vitamins, alcohol, and other poisonous substances in their original containers, locked out of children's sight and reach.
☑ Keep your oven door and dishwasher locked.
☑ Use an appliance lock on the refrigerator, freezer, microwave, trash compacter, and oven.
☑ Plastic wraps and bags should be locked away if they are not tied in knots and discarded.
☑ Store knives and other sharp utensils in drawers or cabinets secured with child-resistant safety latches.
☑ For garbage cans a lock isn't necessary, but they should be kept securely covered and out of the reach of children.

Test It!

☑ Test the tap water in your home for lead, especially if you have an older home.

Do It!

☑ Use back burners and keep pot handles turned to the back of the stove.
☑ Use spill-resistant mugs for hot beverages.
☑ Keep your child in a crib, play yard, or high chair while anyone is cooking, away from the cooking area and away from any wall or counter from which he can push off.
☑ Make sure the floor is nonslip and free of grease. Promptly clean up any spills.

Not!

☑ Never leave your child unsupervised in the kitchen.
☑ Don't use tablecloths or place mats, thus avoiding the risk of your child's pulling a hot beverage or hot food down on herself.
☑ Don't set mugs of hot coffee and other hot foods near the edge of counters or tables.

☑ Do not hold or carry your child while holding hot foods or beverages.

☑ Do not let your child use the microwave.

☑ Never heat a bottle in the microwave.

☑ Don't serve round, firm food.

☑ Never leave any liquid-filled bucket or container unattended.

Do-It-Yourself Safety in the Bathroom

Install It!

☑ Apply a rubber suction bath mat or non-slip strips to the tub and shower.

☑ Install grab bars in the bath and shower.

☑ Attach a securely fitting cushion over the tub spout.

Lock It!

☑ Keep all harmful items that are commonly kept in the bathroom—such as medicine, cosmetics, grooming products, and sharp objects—locked and out of children's reach and sight.

☑ Place safety locks on all toilet lids.

Test It!

☑ Always regulate and test the water before you or your children get into the bathtub or shower.

Do It!

☑ Set the water thermostat to 120°F or lower.

☑ Use a rubber-backed rug on the floor for stepping out of the tub or shower.

☑ Always empty bath water immediately after use.

Not!

☑ Never leave children unattended in the bathroom, even for a few seconds.

☑ Never leave electrical appliances near water or within the reach of your child.

Do-It-Yourself Safety in the Nursery

Do It!

☑ Buy a new crib that meets current safety standards.

☑ Look for the JPMA label—the certification seal from the Juvenile Products Manufacturers Association—when you buy any baby equipment.

☑ Make sure the crib is sturdy, with no loose, broken, missing, or improperly installed hardware.

☑ Position any mobile or hanging crib toy out of your child's reach. Remove any hanging toys when the baby begins to push up on his hands and knees, or when he is 5 months old, whichever comes first.

☑ Avoid strings on infant products, including pacifiers and rattles.

☑ Make sure the crib sheet fits properly. If it is too loose or so tight it pops up from the corner, it can become a strangulation hazard.

☑ Always put your baby on his back to sleep at night and naptime, on a firm, tight-fitting mattress with a crib sheet that fits securely. Remove all soft objects and loose bedding from the sleep area. Bare is best.

Not!

☑ Never hang anything on or above a crib with a string or ribbon longer than 7 inches.

☑ Do not place the crib near windows, draperies, window covering cords, electrical cords, baby monitor cords and other cords, hanging wall decorations, heating sources, or climbable furniture.

Do-It-Yourself Safety in the Living Room and Family Area

Lock It!

☑ Small objects, if not locked away, should be kept out of children's sight and reach.

Test It!

☑ Use an empty toilet paper roll to make certain a toy is not a choking hazard. If the toy fits in the roll, it's not safe.

Do It!

☑ Use hardware-mounted safety gates at the top and bottom of stairs as long as an infant or toddler is in your home.

☑ Keep stairs well lit and clear of clutter; have light switches at both the bottom and the top of the stairway.

☑ Tack down loose carpet edges with carpet tape or tacks.

☑ Identify and remove poisonous house plants.

☑ Buy age-appropriate toys for your child.

☑ Anchor TVs and top-heavy furniture to prevent them from tipping over.

☑ Use corner and edge guards on furniture and fireplace hearths.

Not!

☑ Do not use scatter rugs. If it is necessary to have them, add a nonskid backing or nonskid mat underneath them.

☑ Do not keep furniture (including chairs, benches, tables, toy boxes, or bookcases) near windows, draperies or window covering cords.

Do-It-Yourself Safety in the Garage

Install It!

☑ Install an auto-reverse feature and an entrapment protection feature—such as a photoelectric sensor—to the automatic garage-door opener.

Lock It!

☑ Store and lock poisonous materials out of children's reach.

☑ Store flammable liquids like gasoline in safety-approved containers outside the home, in a well-ventilated, locked shed or detached garage, and away from any source of ignition.

☑ Keep all tools out of children's reach.

Do It!

☑ Empty any bucket right away after use, and store all buckets upside down.

Not!

☑ Never store flammable materials near a heat source.

Do-It-Yourself Safety in the Backyard
Install It!

- ☑ Apply cushioning under playground equipment—either rubber or synthetic mats or loose fill material such as sand, pea gravel, wood products, or loose rubber products at a depth of 12 inches.
- ☑ Place a cover over the sandbox when children are not using it, so that animals cannot use it as a litter box.

Lock It!

- ☑ Securely store lawn equipment and garden tools when they are not in use.
- ☑ After using the barbecue grill, properly lock it away, along with charcoal, propane, and the lighter or matches.

Do it!

- ☑ Enclose the backyard.
- ☑ Remove or fence in all toxic plants.
- ☑ Pull up mushrooms regularly, especially after rainy weather.
- ☑ Keep steps and paved areas clean and well maintained.
- ☑ Promptly clean up animal droppings.
- ☑ Keep your child indoors and supervised at all times when any outdoor power equipment is being used.

Not!

- ☑ Never take a child for a ride on a garden tractor or riding mower.

Do-It-Yourself Safety around Your Home Pool
Install It!

- ☑ Install a 4-sided fence at least 4 feet high, equipped with a self-closing, self-latching gate.

Lock It!

- ☑ Equip all doors with child-resistant locks.
- ☑ Store pool supplies and chemicals locked out of reach of children.

Test It!

- ☑ Inspect pool and equipment regularly.

Do It!

☑ When children are ready, enroll them in a learn-to-swim class taught by qualified instructors.

☑ Make sure all children have constant, undistracted adult supervision when swimming. No child is drownproof.

☑ Keep rescue equipment, emergency numbers, and a phone poolside.

Common Poisonous Plants

Do not assume that if a particular plant does not appear on this list that it is safe. This is not an all-inclusive list. Call the Poison Help line at 800-222-1222 to be sure.

Angels Trumpet (*Datura* species)
Autumn Crocus *(Colchicum autumnale)*
Azalea *(Rhododendron* species)
Black Locust *(Robinia pseudoacacia)*
Caladium *(Caladium* species)
Castor Bean *(Ricinus communis)*
Chokecherry *(Prunus virginiana)*
Climbing, or Deadly, Nightshade *(Solanum dulcamara)*
Daffodil (genus *Narcissus)*
Daphne *(Daphne* species)
Deadly Nightshade, or Belladonna *(Atropa belladonna)*
Delphinium (genus *Delphinium)*
Dumb Cane (genus *Dieffenbachia)*
Elephant Ear *(Colocasia esculenta)*
English Ivy *(Hedera helix)*
Foxglove *(Digitalis purpurea)*
Hyacinth (Hyacinthus orientalis)
Hydrangea *(Hydrangea* species)
Iris (genus *Iris)*
Jack-in-the-Pulpit *(Arisaema triphyllum)*

Jimsonweed *(Datura stramonium)*
Lantana *(Lantana camara)*
Larkspur *(Delphinium* species)
Lily of the Valley *(Convallaria majalis)*
Mayapple *(Podophyllum peltatum)*
Monkshood *(Aconitum napellus)*
Morning Glory (genus *Ipomoea)*
Mountain Laurel *(Kalmia latifolia)*
Oleander *(Nerium oleander)*
Philodendron (genus *Philodendron)*
Poison Hemlock *(Conium maculatum)*
Pokeweed *(Phytolacca americana)*
Privet *(Ligustrum vulgare)*
Rhododendron (genus *Rhododendron)*
Rosary Pea *(Abrus precatorius)*
Sweet Pea *(Lathyrus odoratus)*
Virginia Creeper (Parthenocissus quinquefolia)
Water Hemlock (genus *Cicuta)*
Wisteria (genus *Wisteria)*
Yew (genus *Taxus)*

Holiday Plants

American Mistletoe *(Phoradendron flavescens)*
Christmas Rose *(Helleborus niger)*
European Mistletoe *(Viscum album)*
Holly (genus *Ilex)*
Jerusalem Cherry *(Solanum pseudocapsicum)*

Essential Safety Products and the Do-It-Yourself Shopper

When it comes to safety in your home, you must be the expert. This book empowers you to do that. Like any other expert, you need tools to enable you to do what must be done. This shopping list will allow you to check your supplies and quickly see what you need to purchase. These items can be purchased online, and at hardware stores, baby equipment stores, home improvement stores and supermarkets. Make sure all these items are properly and carefully installed and are well maintained. Please check them frequently. Remember, no child-safety device is completely childproof. Proper supervision is always required.

Tools for Food Safety
- Vegetable scrub brush
- Food thermometers
- Appliance thermometers for refrigerator and freezer (refrigerator, 40°F or below; freezer, 0°F or below)

Tools for Home Safety
- Doorknob covers

- Door locks
- Decals on glass doors
- Door stops and door holders to save precious fingers from being crushed
- Baby monitor

Tools for Fire Safety

- Smoke alarms for every bedroom, outside each separate sleeping area, and on every level of the home, including the basement.
- Flame-resistant or snug-fitting sleepwear for your children (check the label)
- Multipurpose fire extinguishers for kitchen, basement, and work-shop area

Tools for Emergencies

- Fully stocked first aid kit (See chapter 14)
- Form for Emergency Numbers. Post a copy near every telephone, on the refrigerator, and in the safe room. (See Appendix F, "Form for Emergency Numbers.")
- Fully stocked disaster supplies kit, including nonperishable foods, flashlights, batteries, and water
- Cell phone

Tools for the Prevention of Choking, Suffocation, and Strangulation

- Cordless window coverings
- Empty toilet paper roll to make certain a toy is not a choking hazard. If the toy fits in the roll, it's not safe.
- Cord shorteners to eliminate excess electrical cords

Tools for the Prevention of Electrocution

- Ground fault circuit interrupters (GFCIs)
- Electrical outlet safety covers and outlet plates (Be sure outlet plug caps cannot easily be removed by a child and are not a choking hazard.)
- Power strip cover

Tools for the Prevention of Burns

- Guards on stove knobs
- Appliance lock for microwave
- Oven-door lock
- Spill-resistant mug for hot beverages

Tools for the Prevention of Poisoning

- Safety latches and locks for drawers and cabinets
- Child-resistant packaging (remember they are not childproof)
- Carbon monoxide alarms for every sleeping area, on every level of the home and at least 15 feet from any fuel-burning appliances
- Appliance lock for refrigerator

Tools for the Prevention of Falls . . . And Cushions for Falls That Happen

- Window safety devices with quick-release mechanisms for fire exits; check local codes
- Hardware-mounted gates for top and bottom of stairs
- Power-failure nightlights for bedroom, hallways, stairs, and bathrooms
- Corner and edge guards for all sharp edges
- Nonskid backing on all rugs
- Rubber suction bath mat
- Grab bars for bath and shower
- Brackets, braces and wall straps to secure TVs and furniture to the wall
- Cushioned spout cover for bathtub
- Auto-reverse feature on automatic garage-door opener
- Photoelectric sensor or edge sensor on automatic garage door opener
- Cushioning to place under playground equipment: sand, pea gravel, wood products, or loose rubber products for depth of 12 inches; or synthetic or rubber mats

Tools for the Prevention of Drowning

- Pool fence, 4 feet high surrounding all 4 sides and with self-closing, self-latching gates
- Toilet bowl safety lock
- Locked safety cover for spa
- U.S. Coast Guard-approved life preserver, life jackets, and ring buoy with line securely attached, or a long-handled hook to assist or retrieve a victim from the water

Tools for the Prevention of Harm from Firearms in the Home

- Gun locks
- Gun cabinets, vaults, or safes (one place for locking away unloaded firearms, another for locking away ammunition)

Tools for the Prevention of Harm Away from Home

- Reflective tape to be attached to child's outwear when she is out at dawn, dusk, or evening
- Bike helmet, properly fitted, meeting current national guidelines (See Chapter 16, "Traveling with Baby")
- Car safety seat that is correct for your child's age and size and for your particular car (See Chapter 16, "Traveling with Baby")

Recall Information

Recalled products are those that have been found to be unsafe, hazardous, or defective. To provide better service in alerting consumers, the federal government has created one comprehensive recall site to which you may go for all types of recall information: *www.recalls.gov.* The website links visitors to the home pages of government regulatory agencies responsible for product recalls. You may still contact individual government agencies directly.

If you do not choose to visit the recall site on a regular basis, to stay current on this matter you may, instead, subscribe to the site's email notification of recalls. It is important that you, in addition, search through the government agencies' archived information for products you already own. If you discover that a product you own has been recalled, follow the instructions on the recall notice. Report any unsafe product or a product-related injury to the appropriate governmental agency and to the product's manufacturer.

Do not neglect filling out and sending in the registration form that comes with any product, so the company can notify you in the event of a recall. You may also wish to contact individual government agencies for information about specific products. Here's how.

Consumer Products

Agency: CPSC—Consumer Product
   Website: *www.cpsc.gov*
   Hotline: 800-638-2772, staffed M-F 8:00 a.m.-5:30 p.m. EST; messages can be left anytime.
   TTY*: (301) 595-7054
   *Telecommunications device for the deaf

If you have a safety issue with any product, including toys and children's products, you can report it to SaferProducts.gov, a database maintained by the US Consumer Product Safety Commission that allows consumers to report safety issues and research products to see what experiences other consumers have had, even if it has not been recalled.

Motor Vehicles and Related Equipment, Child Safety Seats and Tires

Agency: NHTSA—National Highway Traffic Safety Administration, U.S. Department of Transportation (DOT)
Website: *www.nhtsa.gov* or *www.safercar.gov*
Hotline: 888-DASH-2-DOT [327-4236], staffed M-F 8 a.m.-8 p.m. EST
TTY: 800-424-9153

Boats (Recreational Boats and Related Equipment)

Agency: USCG—U.S. Coast Guard
Website: *www.uscgboating.org*

Food, Medicine and Cosmetics

Agency: FDA—Food and Drug Administration. This agency has jurisdiction over recalls involving the following: Food for human consumption, pet food and animal feed, cosmetics, drugs, vaccines, medical devices, blood and plasma products, other biologics, and veterinary products.
Website: *www.fda.gov*
Hotline: 888-INFO-FDA [463-6332]

Meat and Poultry Products (Including Eggs)

Agency: USDA—U.S. Department of Agriculture, Food Safety and Inspection Service (FSIS).
Website: *www.fsis.usda.gov*
Hotline: 888-MPHOTLINE [674-6854], staffed M-F 10 a.m.-6 p.m. EST
TTY: 800-256-7072

Environmental Products (Pesticides, Rodenticides, Fungicides, Vehicle Emission Testing)

Agency: EPA—Environmental Protection Agency
Website: *www.epa.gov*

Helpful Resources

General Safety

American Academy of Pediatrics: *www.aap.org* and *www.healthychildren.org*

Consumer Products Safety Commission: *www.cpsc.gov* and *www.saferproducts.gov* or (800) 638-2772

National Safety Council: *www.nsc.org* or (800) 621-7615

Safe Kids WorldWide: *www.safekids.org* or (202) 662-0600

Specific Safety Concerns

Air Quality

Environmental Protection Agency, Indoor Air Quality: Go to *www.epa.gov/iaq*

Art Supplies

The Art & Creative Materials Institute, Inc.: *www.acmiart.org* or (781) 556-1044

Bicycle Safety

Bicycle Helmet Safety Institute: Offers information on bicycle helmets. Go to *www.helmets.org* or call (703) 486-0100.

League of American Bicyclists: To locate a class in your area that will teach how to ride a bicycle safely: *www.bikeleague.org* or (202) 822-1333

Breast Feeding

La Leche League International: *www.llli.org/nb.html* or call the help-line (877) 4 LALECHE [452-5324]
Centers for Disease Control and Prevention: *www.cdc.gov /breastfeeding*
The Office on Women's Health, U.S. Department of Health and Human Services: Go to *www.womenshealth.gov/Breastfeeding* or call the helpline (800) 994-9662

Burn Prevention

Burn Prevention Foundation: *www.burnprevention.org* or (610) 969-3930
Children's Burn Foundation: *www.childburn.org* or (800) 949-8898
National Fire Protection Agency: *www.nfpa.org* or (800) 344-3555

Child Care

Child Care Aware: Offers information about child care referral agencies in your area. Go to *www.childcareaware.org* or call (800) 4242246.
National Association for the Education of Young Children (NAEYC): Provides a list of NAEYC-accredited early childhood programs in your area. Go to *www.naeyc.org* or call (800) 424-2460.
National Association for Family Child Care (NAFCC): Offers information regarding accredited family child care in your area. Go to *www.nafcc.org* or call (801) 886-2322.
National Data Base of Child Care Licensing Regulations gives licensing information for states: *childcareta.acf.hhs.gov/licensing*

Child Passenger Safety

American Academy of Pediatrics: *www.aap.org* and *www .healthychildren.org*
National Highway Traffic Safety Administration (NHTSA): *www.nhtsa.gov,* or *www.safercar.gov,* or (888) DASH-2-DOT [327-4236]
Kids and Cars: A national nonprofit organization working to reduce injury and death of children in or around motor vehicles. Visit *www.kidsandcars.org* or call (913) 732-2792.
Safe Kids Worldwide: *www.safekids.org* or (202) 662-0600

SafetyBeltSafe U.S.A.: The national non-profit organization, solely devoted to child passenger safety, works to reduce the number of serious and fatal traffic injuries suffered by children by promoting the correct, consistent use of safety seats and safety belts. Go to *www.carseat.org* or (800) 745-SAFE (7233).

Cribs

Cribs for Kids: Educates health professionals and the public about the safest way an infant should be put down to sleep. In addition to education and infant safe sleep programming, Cribs for Kids provides safe sleeping environments at discounted prices. These products are distributed through a network of over 1,000 partners nationwide. Go to *www.cribsforkids.org*.

Diapers

Real Diaper Association: A nonprofit organization that promotes the use of simple, reusable cloth diapers. To learn more about the advantages of using cloth diapers, go to *www.realdiaperassociation.org*.

Emergency Preparedness

Federal Emergency Management Agency (FEMA): Part of the U.S. Department of Homeland Security. Go to *www.fema.gov* or *www.ready.gov*

The National Oceanic and Atmospheric Administration/National Weather Service (NOAA): *www.nws.noaa.gov*

Energy Saving

U.S Department of Energy: Offers simple ways you can reduce your energy use at home with No-Cost and Low-Cost Tips. Go to *energy.gov/science-innovation/energy-efficiency*.

Fire Safety

National Fire Protection Agency: *www.nfpa.org* or (800) 344-3555
U.S. Fire Administration: *www.usfa.fema.gov*

Firearm Safety

Brady Center to Prevent Handgun Violence: *www.bradycampaign.org* or call (202) 370-8101; Ask Campaign: *www.askingsaveskids.org*
NRA Community Service Program (Eddie Eagle Gun Safety Program): *eddieeagle.nra.org* or (800) 672-3888

Project ChildSafe: Sponsored by the National Shooting Sports Foundation (a non-profit trade association), has distributed 37 million gun lock safety kits. NSSF also provides safety brochures to gun owners and firearm safety videos to schools free of charge. Learn more at *www.nssf.org.*

Fireworks

National Council on Fireworks Safety, Inc.: *www.fireworksafety.com*

Flying

Federal Aviation Administration: *www.faa.gov*

Food Safety

Environmental Protection Agency: Offers advice about high concentrations of chemical contaminates in local fish and wildlife. Go to *www.epa.gov/fish-tech.*

Environmental Working Group: Provides information on mercury in fish and on pesticides and other toxic chemicals in food and water. Go to *www.ewg.org* or *www.foodnews.org.*

Stop Foodborne Illness: A nonprofit organization working to prevent food-borne illnesses. Go to *www.stopfoodborneillness.org.*

USDA/Food Safety and Inspection Service (FSIS): gives information on meat, poultry products and eggs. Go to *www.fsis.usda .gov* or call the Meat and Poultry Hotline (888) MPHOTLINE [674-6854].

Green Products

Forest Stewardship Council: Certifies lumber and forest products that protect forests. Go to *www.fscus.org.*

Home Environment

One way to be confident you are doing your best to limit chemicals in your home is to look for GREENGUARD certification, which attests to a product's having been screened for more than 10,000 chemicals by an independent, third-party organization. The GREENGUARD label assures you the product has met some of the world's most rigorous and comprehensive standards for low emissions of volatile organic compounds (VOCs) into indoor air. GREENGUARD certified products include baby cribs, mattresses, countertops, paints and adhesives, and insulation and wood flooring. Go to *www.greenguard.org.*

Immunizations

Centers for Disease Control and Prevention: *www.cdc.gov/vaccines* or the National Immunization Hotline, (800) CDC-[232]-4636

Insect Repellents

Environmental Protection Agency: *www.epa.gov/insect-repellents*

Internet Hoaxes

To check out whether information you receive is a hoax, go to *www.snopes.com*

Juvenile Products

Kids in Danger: Is a nonprofit organization devoted to protecting children by making children's products safer. Go to *www.kidsindanger.org* or call (312) 595-0649.

Keeping Babies Safe: Is a nonprofit organization that provides education, assistance, advocacy and leadership in the development of safer children's products and practices. Go to *www.keepingbabiessafe.org.*

The Juvenile Products Manufacturers Association (JPMA): *www.jpma.org* or call (856) 638-0420 to learn more about the JPMA Certification program.

Lead Poisoning

Environmental Protection Agency: *www.epa.gov/lead* or (800) 424-LEAD [5323]

Local Food

To find family farms, farmers markets and other sources of sustainably-grown food in your area, go to *www.localharvest.org*

Mosquitos

Centers for Disease Control and Prevention: West Nile Virus, go to *www.cdc.gov/westnile/index*. Zika, go to *www.cdc.gov/zika/index.html.*

Personal Safety

Child Watch of North America: Maintains a 24-hour toll-free hotline for information on missing children. To receive information and find out where you can get free photo ID cards and fingerprinting, go to *www.childwatch.org* or call (888) CHILD-WATCH [244-5392].

National Center for Missing and Exploited Children: Gives and receives information on missing and exploited children 24/7 at *www.missingkids.com* or through its hotline, (800) THE LOST [8435678]

Pesticide Safety/Alternatives

Beyond Pesticides: A a nonprofit organization committed to pesticide safety and the adoption of alternative pest management strategies. Go to *www.beyondpesticides.org* or call (202) 543-5450.

Healthy Child Healthy World: A non-profit organization dedicated to protecting the health and well-being of children from harmful environmental exposures. Visit *www.healthychild.org*.

National Pesticide Information Center: *www.npic.orst.edu* or (800) 858-7378

Playground Safety

National Program for Playground Safety: *www.playgroundsafety.org* or (800) 554-7529

Poison

The Poison Help Line: Provides information about poisons in the home. Call (800) 222-1222, the number for every poison center in the United States. Call this number 24 hours a day, 7 days a week to talk to a poison expert. Call right away if you have a poison emergency. Also call if you have a question about a poison or about poison prevention. Or go to *triage.webpoisoncontrol.org*.

Postpartum Depression/Anxiety

Postpartum Support International (PSI): A non-profit organization dedicated to helping women and men suffering from perinatal mood and anxiety disorders including postpartum depression. Support, resources, and information are free and confidential. Go to *www.postpartum.net* or call (800) 944-4PPD [4773].

Pregnancy

March of Dimes: Offers information about pregnancy, birth defects, genetics, drug and alcohol use, and environmental hazards during pregnancy and other related topics. Go to *www.modimes.org*.

Preventing Tip Overs

Consumer Products Safety Commission: www.anchorit.gov

Product Ratings

Consumer Reports: A nonprofit organization dedicated to empowering you to make informed choices about the products you buy, providing unbiased product ratings and reviews. They put over 5000 products through rigorous testing each year. Go to *www.consumerreports.org*.

Radon

National Radon Program Services Hotline: Allows you to speak to a radon specialist and/or order a low-cost test kit. Call (800) 55-RADON [557-2366].

National Radon Fix-It Line: Helps people whose homes have elevated radon levels by giving guidance for taking the necessary steps toward fixing their homes. Call 800-644-6999.

Restaurants

Healthy Dining Finder: Search for restaurants that provide nutritious options based on criteria such as ZIP code, type of cuisine, and price range. Visit *www.healthydiningfinder.com*.

Safety Training

American Red Cross: Gives information about local chapters and tells which ones offer courses on CPR, water safety, and babysitting at *www.redcross.org*

American Heart Association: Find a CPR course near you, at *www.americanheart.org*

Shaken Baby Syndrome

National Center on Shaken Baby Syndrome: *www.dontshake.org* or (801) 447-9360

Sudden Infant Death Syndrome

First Candle: *www.firstcandle.org* or (800) 221-SIDS [7437]
Pam Borchardt: www.SafeSleepTraining.com

Sun Safety

Environmental Protection Agency: *www.epa.gov/sunsafety*
Centers for Disease Control and Prevention: *www.cdc.gov/cancer /skin/basic_info/children.htm*

Tick-Borne Diseases

American Lyme Disease Foundation: *www.aldf.com*
Centers for Disease Control and Prevention: *www.cdc.gov/ticks /index.html*

Tobacco Smoke

The American Lung Association: Offers free educational material on smoking and lung disease and information on smoking cessation programs in your area. Go to *www.lungusa.org* or call (800) LUNG USA [586-4872].
Centers for Disease Control and Prevention: *www.cdc.gov/tobacco /index.htm*

Travel Abroad

Centers for Disease Control and Prevention: Offers health information for international travelers at *www.cdc.gov/travel*
U.S. Department of State, Bureau of Consular Affairs: Provides information on obtaining passports and visas and offers travel advisories about individual countries. Visit *www.travel.state.gov*.

Tummy Time Tips

American Physical Therapy Association: Offers materials on its web-site that can guide you in positioning and exercising your new baby. Go to *www.apta.org*.
Judy Towne Jennings, PT, MA: A researcher, has several publications about tummy time that can be downloaded from her webpage, *www.fit-baby.com*

Water Quality (drinking water)

Environmental Protection Agency: *www.epa.gov/ground-water-and-drinking-water* or *www.epa.gov/safewater/labs/index.html* or call Hotline (800) 426-4791

International Bottled Water Association: An organization representing the bottled water industry. Go to *www.bottledwater.org* or call (703) 683-5213 or the information hotline (800) WATER-11 [928-3711].

NSF International: Offers information on evaluating filtering devices. Go to *www.nsf.org* or call (734) 769-8010 or (800) NSFMARK [673-6275].

Underwriters Laboratories, Inc.: Tests and certifies home water treatment units; their label is on units, Go to *www.ul.com.*

Water Quality Association: Classifies units according to the contaminants the devices remove, as well as listing units that have earned the organization's "Good Seal" approval. Go to *www.wqa.org* or call (630) 505-0160.

Window Safety

Best for Kids program: Sponsored by the Window Covering Manufacturers Association (WCMA), it is designed to help identify window covering products that are certified as best suited for use in homes with young children. Go to *www.windowcoverings.org.*

Parents for Window Blind Safety (PFWBS): Window coverings that have the PFWBS lab-tested, Mom-approved seal are in stores near you or online. For more information, go to *www.pfwbs.org.*

Form for Emergency Numbers

Use this form to collect all emergency numbers for use in your home. In a crisis situation, it should be handy for you or anyone staying in your home to use. Post a copy near every telephone and on the refrigerator. Post one in the safe room, as well. Program emergency numbers into phones.

Emergency 911 _____

Police _____

Fire Department _____

Ambulance _____

Pediatrician _____

Family doctor _____

Dentist _____

Poison Help line <u>1-800-222-1222</u> _____

Pharmacy _____

Out-of-town family contact _____

Information to Give in Emergencies

Home

Home address (include all cross streets so that directions can be given)

_____

_____

_____

_____

Home phone number _____

Personal information about the child:

Child's name _____

Date of birth_____

Weight _____

Allergies _____

_____

_____

Current medications_____

_____

_____

Medical conditions _____

_____

_____

How to reach family members:

Mom's cell phone and work numbers _____

Dad's cell phone and work numbers _____

Nearest relative or neighbor _____

Phone number _____

TEN STEPS TO
MINDFULNESS MEDITATION

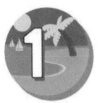

1 Create time & space.
Choose a regular time each day for mindfulness meditation practice, ideally a quiet place free from distraction

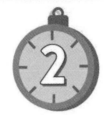

2 Set a timer.
Start with just 5 minutes and ease your way up to 15-40 minutes.

3 Find a comfortable sitting position.
Sit cross-legged on the floor, on the grass, or in a chair your feet flat on the ground.

4 Check your posture.
Sit up straight, hands in a comfortable position. Keep neck long, chin tilted slightly downward, tongue resting on roof of mouth. Relax shoulders. Close eyes or gaze downward 5-10 feet in front of you.

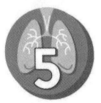

5 Take deep breaths.
Deep breathing helps settle the body and establish your presence in the space

6 Direct attention to your breath.
Focus on a part of the body where the breath feels prominent: nostrils; back of throat; or diaphragm. Try not to switch focus.

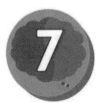

7 Maintain attention to your breath.
As you inhale and exhale, focus on the breath. If attention wanders, return to the breath. Let go of thoughts, feelings or distractions.

8 Repeat steps 6-7.
For the duration of meditation session. The mind will wander. Simply acknowledge this and return to your breath.

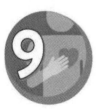

9 Be kind to yourself.
Don't be upset if focus occasionally drifts or if you fall asleep. If very tired, meditate with eyes open and rearrange posture to more erect (but still relaxed) position.

10 Prepare for a soft landing.
When the timer goes off, keep eyes closed until you're ready to open them. Be thankful. Acknowledge your practice with gratitude.

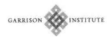

GARRISON INSTITUTE

Index

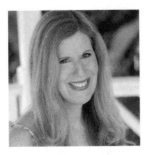

About the Author

Debra Holtzman is a nationally recognized child safety and health expert, specializing in injury prevention, toxic chemicals, food safety, and healthy living. She has been helping families keep their children safe for more than two decades. She has a law degree and an M.A. in occupational health and safety and has worked as a safety and health consultant.

Debra served as a subject matter expert for the American Red Cross "Advanced Child Care" course (StayWell Publishing, April, 2014), and also for the recent version of the American Red Cross "Babysitting Basics" course. She co-wrote the script for the nationally distributed DVD program *Safety Starts at Home: The Essential Childproofing Guide* (InJoy Videos. 2012). She also served as the Content Consultant for the 2012 children's series *Rookie Read-About Safety*, published by Scholastic Books.

She has been a guest on hundreds of broadcast shows, including NBC's *Today Show, Weekend Today, ABC World News*, MSNBC, CNBC, *The Daily Buzz, Bloomberg News*, and *Martha Stewart Living Radio*. Debra has been featured in *Dr. Oz, The Good Life*; CNN; *The New York Times*; *USA Weekend Magazine*; *Parents*; and *Parenting*. She was also the on-camera baby safety expert for the weekly Discovery Health Channel's TV series, "Make Room for Baby."

She was chosen an "Everyday Hero" by *Reader's Digest* and was named a "Woman Making a Difference" by *Family Circle Magazine*. She has served as the Honorary Co-Chair of the Florida Safe Kids Coalition, is a certified child passenger safety technician, and teaches infant and toddler safety and CPR classes at Memorial Regional Hospital in Hollywood, Florida.

Debra lives in South Florida with her husband, Robert, and dog, Rocky. She is the proud mother of Adam and Laura, and is thrilled to be exploring a brand new role—grandmother to baby Emma.

SENTIENT PUBLICATIONS, LLC publishes books on cultural creativity, experimental education, transformative spirituality, holistic health, new science, ecology, and other topics, approached from an integral viewpoint. Our authors are intensely interested in exploring the nature of life from fresh perspectives, addressing life's great questions, and fostering the full expression of the human potential. Sentient Publications' books arise from the spirit of inquiry and the richness of the inherent dialogue between writer and reader.

We are very interested in hearing from our readers. To direct suggestions or comments to us, or to be added to our mailing list, please contact:

SENTIENT PUBLICATIONS
PO Box 7204
Boulder, CO 80304
303-443-2188
contact@sentientpublications.com
www.sentientpublications.com